T0239978

Writing To Improve Healthcare

AN AUTHOR'S GUIDE TO PUBLICATION

Writing To Improve Healthcare

AN AUTHOR'S GUIDE TO PUBLICATION

David P. Stevens, MD

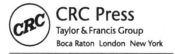

CRC Press
Taylor & Francis Group
Boca Raton London New York

CRC Press is an imprint of the
Taylor & Francis Group, an **informa** business

CRC Press
Taylor & Francis Group
6000 Broken Sound Parkway NW, Suite 300
Boca Raton, FL 33487-2742

International Standard Book Number-13: 978-0-8153-6743-7 (Paperback)
                                       978-0-8153-6744-4 (Hardback)

Visit the Taylor & Francis Web site at
http://www.taylorandfrancis.com

and the CRC Press Web site at
http://www.crcpress.com

Contents

Preface

Healthcare improvement is incomplete until it is published. If there are better, cheaper, safer methods to provide healthcare for patients, it is imperative that those methods be reported—and promptly—to make them available for the benefit of a broad range of patients and health systems. The healthcare improvement work of both practitioners and researchers must find its way to a scholarly literature, just as is required of other healthcare sciences. One would not perform a randomized controlled trial of a new drug and not publish the results. Similarly, one cannot perform innovative healthcare improvement and in conscience not report the results for others. The discovery and sharing of new knowledge that may benefit patients is our reason for working.

The innovations that take place day after day in effective health systems—for example, reduction in waiting times, elimination of avoidable hospital-acquired infections, and medication errors—are successes that need to be spread to all health systems. When health systems fail to provide such care, their patients' care is tacitly—and avoidably—deficient.

This book is intended to speak directly to the large international community of healthcare improvement researchers, educators, and practitioners—physicians, nurses, pharmacists, organization leaders, and their students and trainees.

Foreword

Writing well does not come easily. Most health professionals must work at it early in their training and continue honing writing skills throughout their careers. Sometimes mentors recommend a book on writing. Personally, I still suggest Strunk and White's concise classic *The Elements of Style*, which has stood the test of time as a guide to concise, simple, declarative prose. William Strunk drafted the first version of this classic 100 years ago in 1918 as a teacher of English at Cornell, and was later joined by his co-author and former student, E. B. White (remember *Stuart Little* and *Charlotte's Web*?).

I usually can't resist adding a couple of general tips. The active voice makes writing more engaging and often has the happy effect of shaving off unnecessary length, a frequent goal once manuscripts enter the "revise and resubmit" stage. I also highlight the importance of creating a logical flow from one sentence to the next, as opposed to a series of statements written (or copied and pasted) into an order that reads no better in one sequence compared to another.

The basic tenets of writing joined with a conventional format for the type of research report in question can take an author quite far when it comes to reporting the likes of health services or clinical research. This somewhat prescriptive approach to scientific writing is not necessarily a bad thing, but usually we want strong results to speak for themselves. That said, while we don't want bad writing to get in the way, particularly good writing is not always a dominant goal.

For healthcare improvement authors, by contrast, the writing process often is less formulaic. Writing effectively to accommodate the diverse sciences that underpin healthcare improvement presents fresh challenges. While publication guidelines such as SQUIRE point toward an emerging consensus around relevant elements for such scholarly writing, the nature of improvement work nevertheless pushes authors to broaden the scope of what they might report and emphasize.

A quality improvement report can give rise to a number of different stories. Sometimes, one wants to tell an efficacy story and make a clear case for having successfully addressed a frustrating, widely known problem—improving hand hygiene compliance, for instance, or reducing injurious falls among hospitalized elders. Sometimes how one developed and refined the components of an improvement initiative constitutes the main story. In other cases, the context for the initiative deserves considerable attention along with the associated implementation challenges. And, the story needs to offer lessons for a heterogeneous audience made up of readers from disciplines other than those of the authors, including different healthcare professions and different research traditions, from epidemiology to sociology and psychology. Whatever the story or its elements, it all adds up to a greater premium on quality of writing when it comes to healthcare improvement.

David Stevens never lacks for advice about writing. I first met David in 2010 at a scientific conference in Vancouver. Early in our conversation, he startled me by saying with characteristic aplomb, "I've read most of your published work. You should be an editor." A long story made very short (a common writing objective), I had the honor of succeeding him as editor-in-chief of *BMJ*'s principal journal on healthcare improvement and patient safety as it underwent transformation into *BMJ Quality and Safety*.

Now comes *Writing to Improve Healthcare: An Author's Guide to Publication*. In this book David explores the specific challenges of writing for publication about healthcare improvement and patient safety. He draws on lessons learned from his experiences editing *Quality and Safety in Health Care*—the predecessor journal of *BMJ Quality and Safety*—and his work with resident trainees and faculty in monthly writing sessions at Dartmouth–Hitchcock Medical Center in New Hampshire.

It's my turn to comment on *his* writing. David has learned his lessons well. His emphasis on writing that focuses deeply on the reader, the importance of effective collaboration among co-authors, and strategies that actually employ improvement techniques to improve the writing itself all count as examples of those lessons. Moreover, his focus on publication as an integral part of the work of healthcare improvement places an even greater imperative on the improvement professional to take on writing as a part of the job.

While writing well will not come easily for most healthcare professionals, *Writing to Improve Healthcare* will help. It fills an empty space in the biomedical literature, and it will serve well the aspiring healthcare improvement author as he or she adds writing to the demanding work of improving patient care and healthcare systems.

Kaveh G. Shojania, MD
Editor-in-Chief,
BMJ Quality and Safety
Professor and Vice Chair, Department of Medicine
Director, University of Toronto
Centre for Quality Improvement and Patient Safety
Toronto, Ontario
January 2018

About the author

David P. Stevens, MD, is editor emeritus of *BMJ Quality and Safety*, having served six years as editor-in-chief of its predecessor journal, *Quality and Safety in Health Care*. In addition, he is adjunct professor at the Dartmouth Institute for Health Policy and Clinical Practice, Lebanon, NH, and senior fellow at the Institute for Healthcare Improvement, Boston, MA. He has published extensively in healthcare improvement and patient safety, conducted national writing workshops and web-based programs as well as an innovative writing program for residents and faculty at Dartmouth–Hitchcock Medical Center—all of which serve as test beds for the strategies advanced in *Writing to Improve Healthcare*. He is a founding member of the SQUIRE Publication Guidelines design team and the author of over 100 peer-reviewed scholarly publications. Earlier in his career he was the Scott R. Inkley Professor of General Internal Medicine and Vice Dean for Academic Affairs at Case Western Reserve School of Medicine, Cleveland, OH. He later served in Washington, DC, as health policy advisor to the chair, U.S. Senate Labor Committee; chief academic affiliations officer for the U.S. Veterans Health Administration; and vice president for Healthcare Improvement for the Association of American Medical Colleges.

Acknowledgments

I am indebted to the many trainees and faculty colleagues who participated in a variety of writing activities with me over the last decade. The most rigorous road testing for the concepts advanced in this book occurred during 6 years of monthly writing seminars that I conducted with resident trainees and faculty in the Healthcare Improvement Writing Program for the Leadership and Preventive Medicine Residency (LPMR) at Dartmouth–Hitchcock Medical Center (D-HMC). The principal aim of the LPMR is to train physicians in population health and organizational leadership for health systems improvement. The residency places a high priority on scholarly publication. These trainees and their faculty were relentless—often appropriately skeptical—with their questions, constructive criticism, and advice that resulted in the refinement of ideas about scholarly writing for healthcare improvement. I am grateful to Paul Batalden who established this unique preventive medicine residency and invited me to develop the writing program. Thank you also to Tina Foster who continues to provide tireless leadership as residency program director.

Practical strategies were also refined in writing conferences in other settings, most notably a multi-institutional writing collaborative underwritten by The Cystic Fibrosis Foundation to prepare a supplement on CF improvement work for *BMJ Quality and Safety*. Bruce Marshall and Kathryn Sabadosa patiently supported and led me through the amazing work of their colleagues in the Cystic Fibrosis Care Network.

A perspective for this book was developed while I was editor-in-chief of the *BMJ* journal, *Quality and Safety in Health Care* (now *BMJ Quality and Safety*). Kaveh Shojania and Mary Dixon-Woods, as my successors as editor-in-chief and deputy editor-in-chief at *BMJ Quality and Safety,* have served as remarkably generous reviewers, teachers, and mentors.

Rita Charon and Kathryn Kirkland patiently led me through the wise reflections that are at the heart of Narrative Medicine. Greg Ogrinc, Louise Davies, and Frank Davidoff have served as co-mentors during monthly SQUIRE-focused conference calls, which have contributed to my sense of the complexity of writing to improve healthcare.

Thank you to the legion of anonymous journal reviewers who contributed immeasurable value to my published articles, making them readable and critical. Like all our colleagues who have seen their work published in scholarly journals, I get to take the credit for your hours of advice and improvement.

I am grateful to Joanna Koster, my editor and publisher at CRC Press, for noticing the promise of this little text. Lisa Rubenstein and Tom Janisse provided enormously useful and supportive reviews of an early manuscript proposal.

Finally, thank you to Don Berwick, Maureen Bisognano, Goran Henricks, and Jennifer Stevens for generous counsel, perspective and humor, and to my wise friend, most critical reader, and wife, Maxine.

CHAPTER 1
The imperative to publish healthcare improvement

HEALTHCARE IMPROVEMENT IS INCOMPLETE UNTIL IT IS PUBLISHED

The goal of the sciences that contribute to improving healthcare is to study, validate, and disseminate the new knowledge that is discovered in improvement initiatives. The ultimate aim of this work must be to make that new knowledge available for the benefit of all patients and health systems. In a word, healthcare improvement is incomplete until it is published.

This book is about *your* writing—the complex process that leads to your improvement work's publication. To that end, we will explore the many moving parts and interfaces that are found between your first draft and your ultimate goal, a patient's better care.

Publication also holds your work up to scrutiny by other colleagues who are committed to improving patient care too. Moreover, precious healthcare resources require that improvement work be published so that others, perhaps unaware of your results, do not unknowingly and unnecessarily duplicate it.

Healthcare improvement authors—from novices to experts—find writing for publication challenging in large measure because healthcare improvement science is a constantly evolving scholarly field. This is no more difficult than scholarly writing for other biomedical sciences. Nevertheless successful publication requires a defined strategy. The aim of this book is to provide you an understanding of such a strategy for your own success.

1

This evolving science goes by many names, and will be found in different institutional niches. The institutional leadership where you work to improve healthcare may have decided to call it healthcare improvement, or implementation science or healthcare delivery science. The underlying principles of improving patient care can also be found in health services research that is performed in traditional clinical or basic sciences departments. The important role played by the social sciences must be emphasized here as well. Earnest quasi-ecclesiastical academic arguments have emerged about what is the one, true discipline that "owns" healthcare improvement. As much as possible, we will avoid taking a position in these discussions. Patients and health systems will be best served by our exploration of how and where these fields converge.

Now, a comment about what this book is *not*. While we will probe effective *writing* about improvement, this is not a primer on healthcare improvement or health services research *methodology*. Our approach primarily is to focus on preparing the manuscript that best describes your unique improvement initiative, and your critical interpretation of what and how it happened.

THIS IS DIFFERENT FROM WRITING FOR MOST BIOMEDICAL FIELDS

This is about more than "look what we did." It is about "this is what we did, how we did it, and this is how you, the reader, can do it as well." This is in spite of the fact that your setting and context and that of your reader are inevitably quite different.

Moreover, there are other differences in this approach to writing compared to the experience you may have had writing for other biomedical fields. At its core, healthcare improvement science explores the complex social processes that are found in efforts to change individual and institutional practices. It must accommodate a deep understanding of how each new setting—the context—provides substantial drivers as well as barriers to potentially successful replication of your initiative. It also calls for communicating statistical methods that can validate your results. This statistical methodology will frequently be unfamiliar to many biomedical scientists including editors and reviewers.

Moreover, there is urgency to writing and publishing your healthcare improvement work. I have a colleague who believes that the unfolding pace of time in academic institutions differs depending on your perspective. He is convinced that "academic medicine time" is slower than "the real time of patient needs." In any event, effective and timely communication of valid healthcare improvement strategies is imperative. For example, reduction in waiting times, elimination of central intravenous line infections, and reduction in medical errors are successes that need to be spread to all health systems. Every day that a patient is cared for in a setting that does not provide safe and effective care is an avoidable failure in that patient's personal healthcare.

IMPROVEMENT PROCESSES THAT CAN FACILITATE YOUR WRITING

You will find that there are strategies that you can readily adapt from your healthcare improvement experience that will contribute to your writing effectiveness and efficiency. For example, be attentive to approaches that eliminate wasteful and repetitious processes. One such approach that many improvement authors have found useful is to begin a manuscript simultaneously with the beginning of an improvement initiative. This seemingly unconventional approach—writing before the innovation is fully developed and implemented—offers many efficiencies including the opportunity for ongoing critical reflection on the draft manuscript as it proceeds alongside the improvement initiative (see Chapter 2).

Additional improvement strategies include application of high performance microsystem concepts to facilitate efficient work with your co-authors, and writing in formal writing collaboratives to enhance individual writing quality and productivity. Furthermore, at its foundation, rigorous peer review is in fact a systematic improvement process akin to classical Plan-Do-Study-Act cycles. We will explore in detail each of these concepts in later chapters.

DEVELOP YOUR OWN ROADMAP TO SUCCESSFUL PUBLICATION

Now, a few words about how you can make the best use of this book to facilitate your successful writing for publication. You do not need to start at the beginning of the book and plow through chapter by chapter. Take a look at the table of contents to determine if you want to jump about in your reading to create the sequence of chapters that is most useful to your own writing. For example, you might want to go straight to Chapter 6 to develop

your own personal context for more efficient and productive writing. Or—
if you are like me, and truth be told, prefer to visualize more concretely
where you are headed—you may want to go straight to Chapter 9 for an
effective process for submitting your manuscript to a journal.

You might consider another approach based on Table 1.1. Here
you will find a summary of learning goals that were described by

Table 1.1 Learning goals reported by international participants in a
series of diverse writing seminars and courses

Learning Goal	In which chapter might you specifically find this discussed?
1. Writing for publication is very frustrating—I don't feel like I have anything new or innovative to write.	1, 2, 3, 7, 8
2. Scholarly writing is my weakest area. I find it hard to do it. But it is required in academia for promotion and tenure so I am here to make my scholarly writing better.	1, 2, 5, 7–9
3. Capture specific tools to improve writing in general.	2, 3, 5, 7–9
4. Learn how to get my paper accepted.	2, 9
5. To find inspiration.	1, 6
6. We are working on lots of important projects in our department, so I need to know how I can publish them to increase the impact of these projects.	2, 3, 4, 9
7. I want to evaluate a current draft paper for its likely publication.	2, 5, 7–9
8. Explore journal options for publication.	9
9. Get into a mental framework with discipline to start writing more consistently.	2, 6
10. Learn content and format for publishing.	2, 7–9
11. Learn how and where to publish my improvement work.	2, 9

(Continued)

Table 1.1 (*Continued*) Learning goals reported by international participants in a series of diverse writing seminars and courses

Learning Goal	In which chapter might you specifically find this discussed?
12. Publish more.	2, 3, 9
13. Find journals that publish my kind of research.	9
14. I have not published before and would like to learn strategies and guidelines to do so.	1, 2, 9
15. Learn how to report statistical data.	8
16. Learn how to move from clinical publishing to improvement work and supporting others who should be publishing their work.	1, 2, 7–9
17. New to scholarly writing in general.	1–3
18. Learn to seek out a project that will likely be publishable.	1
19. How, where to publish a paper on our experience with cultural transformation.	2–4, 7–9
20. Lots of energy around improvement—want to reinforce QI as a scholarly pursuit and reinforce benefits of faculty involvement in QI.	1, 2, 6–9
21. To overcome my busy schedule and publish more.	6
22. Identify targets for improvement publication (versus scientific paper writing).	9
23. A more systematic approach to preparing our work for publication.	2, 4, 6–9
24. How can SQUIRE help us edit drafts?	2
25. More strategic approach to reviewing.	5
26. What's different about the scholarly improvement literature?	1, 2, 7–9

colleagues—an international collection of aspiring authors from diverse healthcare professions—who participated in writing workshops, conferences, and webinars. Many participants had published successfully in other scholarly fields, but they all came to improvement writing as a new endeavor. Take a glance to see what looks familiar. Consider jumping directly to the parts of the book where your own learning goals are specifically addressed—not really an index, more like a roadmap.

HOW DID HEALTHCARE WRITING AND PUBLICATION ARRIVE HERE?

Review of the saga of the emergence of healthcare improvement science—with particular emphasis on writing about it effectively—can provide a foundation for your own work as an author.

Early attention to health system dysfunction was marked by the publication of two groundbreaking reports from the Institute of Medicine (IOM) of the U.S. National Academies of Science. These reports described extensive health system deficiencies along with the associated high prevalence of patient harm that was found in U.S. healthcare settings. The reports attracted the attention of healthcare system leaders and health professionals, but they also resonated with patients who recognized their substantial stake in their own safety and health improvement.

The first report published in 2000, *To Err is Human: Building a Safer Health System*, documented that 44,000 to 98,000 patients died annually in the United States as a consequence of medical errors that occurred during the course of their hospitalization [1]. The second IOM report, published in March 2001, *Crossing the Quality Chasm: A New Health System for the 21st Century*, went further and identified even more extensive healthcare system dysfunction [2]. The earlier errors report was anchored solidly in data, while the later report, also evidence-based, was even more aspirational in nature. *Crossing the Quality Chasm* highlighted the complex social and cultural aspects of healthcare. It proposed a comprehensive and ambitious aim of making the system "safe, effective, patient-centered, timely, efficient, and equitable."

A Harvard pediatrician, Don Berwick, was seminal in framing early healthcare improvement as a *social movement*. As founding CEO of the Boston-based Institute for Healthcare Improvement (IHI), he campaigned early and eloquently [3] for dissemination of healthcare innovation. He championed strategies described in the classical work of Everett Rogers [4]. Berwick's ability to capture the stories of healthcare improvement in articles and speeches has been a thread that weaves through the narrative of evolving healthcare improvement over ensuing years.

AN EMERGING CROSS CURRENT: CALLS FOR METHODOLOGIES BASED ON EVIDENCE

In the first decade of the twenty-first century, a noteworthy cross current emerged in the scholarly healthcare literature. It reflected a concern among some observers that healthcare improvement might be veering off a critical scientific path. Early on, Shojania and colleagues [5] asserted that valid healthcare improvement methodology, particularly its application to improving patient safety, required a critical foundation based on evidence. Thereafter, Auerbach et al. [6] called for greater attention to aligning healthcare improvement with rigorous health services research methodology. They began to insist on an author's obligation to demonstrate validity and reliability.

In an extensive systematic literature review, Greenhalgh and colleagues [7] probed deeply the complexity of the critical social processes that are required to adapt innovations widely across institutions. In work that was commissioned by the UK Department of Health as part of the National Health Service modernization agenda at the time, they described a spectrum of methodologies. These methodologies extended across research traditions and progressed from passive spread (diffusion), to active, planned efforts at spread (dissemination), and directed, intentional efforts at spread of an innovation (implementation). They employed citation technology as well as an exhaustive snowball search methodology that elicited additional sources among primary references,

In the course of this far-reaching work, Greenhalgh et al. developed a "meta-narrative" analytic technique to compensate for what they considered a paucity of rigor that characterized many of the studies. They applied innovative adjustments for the wide heterogeneity of research methodologies. Suffice to say, this extensive work laid a significant theoretical and methodological foundation for the development of dissemination research that would follow.

These several threads converged when editors, health service researchers, information systems experts, as well as clinicians and health systems managers came together in a hotel conference room in Washington DC, in 2005. The meeting was convened by a group of U.S. federal agencies, international medical journals, and public foundations. The sponsors included the Agency for Healthcare Research and Quality (AHRQ), the U.S. Veterans Administration (VA), National Institutes of Health (NIH), Robert Wood Johnson Foundation, and several biomedical journals, including most prominently the *BMJ*.

The conference, *Expanding Research and Evaluation Designs to Improve the Science Base for Health Care and Public Health Quality Improvement* provided a setting for a series of insightful presentations—observations and proposals—and heralded a growing consensus surrounding improvement science. This report provides a useful perspective of the early threads that started in 2005 and would eventually converge as an evolving science [8]. Most relevant to our purposes here as potential authors, the participants began an examination of what a scholarly literature might look like for this new field.

Soon thereafter, Rubenstein and colleagues employed a consensus process with the aim of developing a typology for the healthcare improvement scholarly literature, as it existed at that time. This study surveyed most of the authors, editors, and researchers who had participated in the Washington meeting. They identified 80 published articles that they considered representative of the field at this time.

The survey defined four broad categories of so-called Quality Improvement Interventions (QII). They grouped QII into "(I) empirical literature on development and testing of QIIs, (II) QII stories, theories, and frameworks, (III) QII literature synthesis and meta-analysis, and (IV) development and testing of QII related tools…" [9]. This typology provided a broad perspective on which authors, editors, and reviewers would proceed to build.

In spite of this organizing framework, there existed only a handful of journal editors who welcomed healthcare improvement submissions. Two pioneering editors, Fiona Moss and Richard Thomson, had earlier anticipated the importance of Rubenstein's concept of stories, theories, and frameworks by describing editorial expectations for healthcare improvement reports. Their proposal had been published in the nascent bimonthly journal, *Quality in Healthcare* [10], and defined a format for what they called Quality Improvement Reports (QIR). The QIR format was employed in some 50 published improvement reports, principally in *BMJ*-sponsored journals [Koplan KE, 2008, unpublished].

Soon after, there emerged an initiative that called for authors of improvement reports to go beyond a *description* of the improvement intervention. This perspective argued for the *study* of the intervention. With support from the Robert Wood Johnson Foundation, an early draft proposal [11,12] underwent refinement by a formal consensus process among improvement professionals, editors, and authors. The outcome was the early Standards for QUality Improvement Reporting Excellence (SQUIRE) [13].

The elements that were incorporated in the SQUIRE publication guidelines placed strong emphasis on study of the intervention itself—its rationale, methods and outcomes. It highlighted the requirement for a clearly defined study question. It called for critical measurement of an initiative's associated outcomes and the added burden of confidence provided by appropriate statistical methodology. This burden acknowledged the heterogeneity of possible clinical study settings where an improvement initiative might be conducted [14]. This last element—*heterogeneous clinical study settings*—represented substantial divergence from statistical convention in biomedical research [15]. Simply stated, it required statistical methodology that established that the reported outcome *was indeed a result of the initiative* and not a result of confounders in the same clinical setting.

Editors of five journals that principally focused on healthcare improvement reports published and adopted the SQUIRE publication guidelines in 2008. Over time, additional general clinical journals, many in medicine, nursing, and healthcare management, gradually began to accept healthcare improvement submissions.

ANOTHER DEFINING CROSS CURRENT: HUMAN SUBJECTS PROTECTION AND HEALTHCARE IMPROVEMENT

Another defining issue that emerged during the first decade of the twenty-first century was the unique role for human subjects protection in this emerging science. Human subjects protection policy in the United States was driven by government oversight that followed a long and sometimes checkered history regarding human subjects protection in clinical studies. The Hastings Center provided a valuable convening role in the development of consensus around the ethical questions that were raised by healthcare improvement science [16].

Scholarly journals require authors to demonstrate institutional review for studies that involve human subjects. Institutional governance committees, so-called Human Ethics Committees (Institutional Review Boards [IRBs] in the United States), are charged with the important societal role of protecting the safety and welfare of human subjects in clinical research studies.

The Office for Human Research Protections (OHRP), a U.S. federal oversight agency, was formally established in 2000. At that time, OHRP policy considered healthcare improvement studies to be under the rubric of clinical research. Improvement professionals, on the other hand, argued that healthcare improvement did not involve new experimental therapy, but rather the implementation of variations on "usual care" [17]. The variety of approaches to quality improvement at this time employed a variety of definitions of improvement methodology. This added to the conflict surrounding research ethics policy at both the local institutional levels and at the national oversight levels.

The first decade of the twenty-first century was marked by bureaucratic turmoil in IRB policy. In the United States, the standard for human subjects ethical decision-making had been guided historically by a policy known as the Common Rule. Consequently, healthcare improvement professionals faced a challenging period as they tried to fit healthcare improvement studies into the framework defined by the Common Rule [18].

Fortunately for both authors and patients, significant changes in U.S. governmental IRB policy have evolved as it has become increasingly recognized that there are substantial differences between studies that involve human subjects for new therapies as compared to healthcare improvement studies [19]. The defining issue had come to be centered on whether the specific change under study is an acknowledged new therapy, or whether, as in the case of healthcare improvement, it represented the introduction of changes in care that are intended for all patients and if not implemented would result in a poorer standard of care for all.

A substantial federal bureaucratic process—here abbreviated and consequently over-simplified—resulted in a newly drafted "Common Rule" by a widely diverse collection of U.S. federal agencies. Fortunately, a principal outcome of this new formal definition was a revised policy that provided healthcare improvement professionals practical opportunities to seek IRB approval for limited review of human subjects initiatives. The revised policy provides for formal waiver of many of the previous IRB bureaucratic hurdles so long as patient confidentiality issues are specifically addressed [19]. Thus, IRB policy, which had been a particularly thorny issue for improvement professionals, has evolved to a workable solution for the benefit of both patients and improvement professionals.

PUBLICATION GUIDELINES AND IMPROVEMENT WRITING: SQUIRE, STARI, PRISMA, CONSORT, SRQR

Return once more to the topic of the publication guidelines that surround various healthcare improvement formats and methodologies. The first reaction of many authors upon encountering publication guidelines is often, "Spare me! Not more guidelines!" Burdened with guidelines seemingly for every aspect of health system governance and patient care, the last thing that most health professionals want to hear about is yet another set of guidelines.

The good news here is that publication guidelines provide a growing consensus among authors and editors about editorial expectations. To this end, there are a handful of publication guidelines that journal editors have increasingly expected authors to consider as they draft their manuscripts for publication. Acronyms abound in the publication guidelines field, and the list seems to be ever expanding.

CONSORT (Consolidated Standards of Reporting Trials) [20] is a widely accepted standard for reports of randomized controlled trials. There are guidelines that can be particularly useful for healthcare improvement science authors. In addition to SQUIRE, the list includes PRISMA (Preferred Reporting Items for Systematic Reviews and Meta-Analyses) for systematic reviews [21], StaRI (Standards for Reporting Implementation Studies) [22], a useful checklist for elements of implementation science reports, and SRQR (Standards for Reporting Qualitative Research) [23] for reports of qualitative studies. It is important to recognize, however, that publication guidelines are not intended as rigid rules, but as roadmaps for the essential elements in a manuscript—generally a useful consensus that addresses the "what" and "where" of manuscript elements.

After 7 years of road testing by authors, editors, and reviewers, SQUIRE has been revised further by another consensus process and published as version 2.0 [24]. The Guidelines were published simultaneously in 12 journals. Noting this provides a gauge of the evolution of healthcare improvement publication over 7 years—a relatively short time, but a long way from that seminal gathering of editors, improvement scholars, and authors in Washington DC a decade earlier. It suggests that your improvement innovation is ever more likely to find a journal-home, so long as your report adds measurable value for your readers and their patients and health systems.

Finally, the EQUATOR (Enhancing the QUAlity and Transparency of Health Research) network website [25] is the acknowledged authoritative clearinghouse for publication guidelines. It provides a rich source of advice regarding guidelines as well as other useful elements for scholarly writing. As of this writing, the EQUATOR site acknowledges over 350 separate publication guidelines. Needless to say, how you pick among them for useful elements will depend of course on their utility for the study you intend to report.

CONTINUALLY TRACK THE EVOLVING SCIENCE OF HEALTHCARE IMPROVEMENT

The science that underlies your writing—how we know what we know—continues to evolve constantly. Continually tracking this evolution will contribute substantially to your success as a writer. For example, the increasingly permeable boundaries between healthcare improvement science, health services research, and the social sciences further contributes to this diversity. Your mindfulness of such distinctions is important from a theoretic perspective, but pragmatically they offer an ever-expanding source of publication opportunities.

A useful source for tracking the evolution of healthcare improvement science is readily available in the editorial standards of the increasingly diverse scholarly healthcare improvement and patient safety journals—generally found in journals' "Instructions to Authors." An additional handle on this can be provided by regularly reviewing the tables of contents of the same journals.

Strive to expand your network of healthcare improvement colleagues as another source of emerging trends. Specifically pursue the perspectives of colleagues who are members of journal editorial boards.

Regularly review the agendas of scientific sessions at prominent international healthcare improvement meetings and forums. Examples include the *BMJ*/IHI-sponsored International Forum in Europe, the annual IHI National Forum in Orlando, FL, and the annual meeting of the International Society for Quality in Health Care. Similar regional conferences take place in the Middle East, Latin America, and Asia.

A widening community of improvement science-focused researchers now participate in healthcare delivery science sessions at annual health services research conferences. Examples include the annual meetings of AcademyHealth, the U.S. Agency for Healthcare Quality and Research (AHRQ), and specialty societies such as the Academy of Pediatrics, the American Thoracic Society, and the American College of Surgeons.

One more source is the readily available online resources that are devoted to timely collation of the current patient safety literature. Two examples are The Health Foundation (UK) Patient Safety Resource Center [26] and the AHRQ-sponsored Patient Safety Network (PSNet) [27].

This is probably a good place to get started with your actual writing, which we will do in the next chapter.

REFERENCES

1. Kohn LT, Corrigan J, Donaldson MS. (2000). *To Err is Human: Building a Safer Health System*. Washington DC: National Academy Press.
2. Crossing the Chasm Committee on Quality Health Care in America, Institute of Medicine. (2001). *Crossing the Quality Chasm: A New Health System for the 21st Century*. Washington DC: National Academy Press.
3. Berwick DM. Disseminating innovations in healthcare. *JAMA* 2003;289:1969–1975.
4. Rogers E. (1995). *Diffusion of Innovations*. New York, NY: Free Press.
5. Greenhalgh T, Robert G, Macfarlane F, Bate P, Kyriakidou O. Diffusion of innovations in service organizations: Systematic review and recommendations. *Milbank Q* 2004;581–629.

6. Shojania KG, Duncan BW, McDonald KM, Wachter RM. Safe but sound: Patient safety meets evidence-based medicine. *JAMA* 2002;288:508–513.

7. Auerbach AD, Landefeld CS, Shojania KG. The tension between needing to improve care and knowing how to do it. *N Eng J Med* 2007;357:608–613.

8. *Expanding Research and Evaluation Designs to Improve the Science Base for Health Care and Public Health Quality Improvement*, Washington DC, 13–15 September 2005. https://www.hsrd.research.va.gov/quality 2005/. Accessed February 9, 2018.

9. Rubenstein LV, Hemple S, Farmer MM, Asch SM, Yano EM, Dougherty D, Shekelle PW. Finding order in heterogeneity: Types of quality improvement intervention publications. *Qual Saf Health Care* 2008;17:403–408.

10. Moss F, Thomson RG. A new structure for quality improvement reports. *Qual Health Care* 1999:8:76.

11. Davidoff F, Batalden P. Toward stronger evidence on quality improvement. Draft publication guidelines: The beginning of a consensus project. *Qual Saf Health Care* 2005;14:319–325.

12. Stevens DP. Why new guidelines for reporting improvement research? And why now? *Qual Saf Health Care* 2005;14:314.

13. Davidoff F, Batalden P, Stevens D, The SQUIRE study group. Publication guidelines for quality improvement in health care: Evolution of the SQUIRE project. *Qual Saf Health Care* 2008;17 (Suppl 1) i3–i9.

14. Batalden PB, Davidoff F. What is "quality improvement" and how can it transform health care. *Qual Saf Health Care* 2007;16:2–3.

15. Davidoff F. Heterogeneity is not always noise: Lessons from improvement. *JAMA* 2009;302(23):2580–2586.

16. Lynn J, Baily MA, Bottrell M, et al. The ethics of using quality improvement methods in health care. *Ann Intern Med* 2007;146:666–673.

17. Code of Federal Regulations 45 CFR 46 Protection of Human Subjects, 2009. https://www.hhs.gov/ohrp/regulations-and-policy/regulations/45-cfr-46/index.html. Accessed February 9, 2018.

18. Ogrinc G, Nelson WA, Adams SM, O'Hara AE. An instrument to differentiate between clinical research and quality improvement. *IRB: Ethics and Human Research* 2013;35:1–8.

19. Revisions to the Common Rule, 2017. https://www.hhs.gov/ohrp/regulations-and-policy/regulations/finalized-revisions-common-rule/index.html. Accessed February 9, 2018.

20. Schulz KF, Altman DG, Moher D, for the CONSORT Group. CONSORT 2010 Statement: Updated guidelines for reporting parallel group randomized trials. *Ann Int Med* 2010;152:1–7.

21. Moher D, Liberati A, Tetzlaff J, Altman DG, The PRISMA Group. Preferred reporting items for systematic reviews and meta-analyses: The PRISMA statement. *PLoS Med* 2009;6(7):e1000097. PMID: 19621072.

22. Pinnock H, Barwick M, Carpenter CR, et al. Standards for reporting implementation studies. *BMJ* 2017;356:i6795. doi:101136/bmj.i6795.

23. O'Brien BC, Harris IB, Beckman TJ, Reed DA, Cook DA. Standards for reporting qualitative research: A synthesis of recommendations. *Acad Med* 2014;89(9):1245–1251.

24. Ogrinc G, Davies L, Goodman D, Batalden P, Davidoff F, Stevens D. SQUIRE 2.0: Revised publication guidelines from a detailed consensus process. *BMJ Quality and Safety* 2015; Published online first September 2015. doi:10.1136/bmjqs-2015.

25. Enhancing the QUAlity and Transparency of health Research. http://www.equator-network.org/hhh. Accessed February 9, 2018.

26. The Health Foundation Patient Safety Resource Center. http://patientsafety.health.org.uk/. Accessed June 2, 2017.

27. AHRQ Patient Safety Network. https://psnet.ahrq.gov. Accessed February 9, 2018.

CHAPTER 2
Writing to improve healthcare: Preparation of a scholarly manuscript

WRITING FOR HEALTHCARE IMPROVEMENT IS DIFFERENT

"This is not currently written as a scientific article... Nothing is specific. What are registries? ...How are indicators measured? Very vague..." Nearly a decade ago I received this review in response to a journal submission. It was the shortest review I ever encountered (here edited to accommodate journal privacy policy). I suspect you might identify with my reaction. *How did this colleague miss the entire point of my paper?*

On reflection several weeks later, when I had finally retrieved it from the bottom of my inbox, I recognized that my reviewer had implicitly provided the gift of a far more appropriate question. *How did I so completely waste this opportunity to provide a sensible, meaningful manuscript?*

While scholarly writing is challenging for all authors who aspire to publication, writing to improve healthcare holds particular challenges that are different from those for other biomedical topics. In this chapter, we will focus specifically on the basic processes for effective healthcare improvement writing—when to start your manuscript, how to take advantage of reflection that is a part of both writing about healthcare improvement and implementation of the improvement initiative, how to organize your paper, and how to make effective use of selected publication guidelines as an adjunct to effective writing. We will explore in later chapters additional writing strategies for writing efficiency when we explore the imperative to develop a writing style that focuses on your intended reader and working with co-authors.

BEGIN YOUR MANUSCRIPT EARLY

Sitting down and getting started, fully focused, on your manuscript at hand is one of the most daunting moments in writing. The conventional approach to this issue for biomedical research publication is of course to draft the manuscript when the research is finished and the data have been analyzed. In contrast, I urge you to start your draft healthcare improvement manuscript early as you initiate your improvement project.

Wait a minute! How can you possibly write about an initiative that is not even close to completion? We will explore the basic structure outline for your paper in the next section—Introduction, Methods, Results, and Discussion (IMRaD). With the IMRaD structure at hand, this approach to an early start on your manuscript is not as unconventional as it might seem. For example, a draft Introduction can readily be crafted around your systematic literature review. Or a draft Discussion might anticipate the expected outcomes, and will of course evolve over time. In practical terms, your emerging draft will reflect the status of your initiative's results that have been accomplished at each stage of your paper's revision. Both the improvement initiative and the writing processes go forward in tandem, offering unique advantages and efficiencies, and leveraging time for both. As improvement results and the paper's revisions emerge, both processes benefit from classical Plan-Do-Study-Act improvement cycles that unfold in parallel.

EAT DESSERT FIRST

A sign on the wall of the popular bakery/restaurant in Cambridge, MA, *Flour*, reads, "Make life sweeter... eat dessert first." When getting started with a paper for publication, there is no need to craft your draft in the outlined sequence that your journal reader will eventually find. You may have several innovative ideas that simply must get onto a page or screen. Start there. The most challenging times can seem to be when ideas are not fully formed, and they are particularly difficult to move from imagination to paper. Jot down the principal ideas when they arise as the improvement work emerges. Be patient and wait to organize the elements of revisions in later steps, aggregating them—labeling, cutting, and pasting—by topic or theme in the manuscript's IMRaD sections, which we discuss in detail next.

INTRODUCTION, METHODS, RESULTS, AND DISCUSSION (IMRAD), A FAMILIAR STRUCTURE

The IMRaD framework—Introduction, Methods, Results, and Discussion—is a recognizable framework for most scientific papers. It works here as well. You will want to anchor your writing process for a healthcare improvement manuscript in an outline of this same IMRaD design, but it is useful to recognize how healthcare improvement science and other biomedical science papers might play this theme in somewhat different keys.

One useful strategy as you organize your early drafts is to consider publication guidelines as a content checklist. Guidelines offer shared expectations for authors, editors, and reviewers alike. The SQUIRE 2.0 Guidelines [1] provide a useful adjunct, offering in detail the appropriate elements of a scholarly improvement report with in depth guidance for meeting the field's standards of science and scholarship. StaRI (Standards for Reporting Implementation Studies) [2] also offers a useful checklist for explicitly designed implementation science reports.

While the most recent SQUIRE 2.0 Publication Guidelines were published in *BMJ Quality and Safety* [1], the report was also published simultaneously in a dozen other journals whose editors indicated their willingness to consider healthcare improvement submissions.

A particularly useful additional resource is the "Explanation and Evaluation" report that accompanies most formal publication guidelines such as SQUIRE 2.0 [3]. It offers a wealth of useful advice for the author by highlighting previously published papers that provide selected examples of specific SQUIRE elements. Our focus here, however, is to emphasize the overall organization of your report. In that sense, the use of Guidelines at this point in your drafting and revision processes should serve you more as an adjunct rather than the central focus [4].

A good rule is to use Guidelines specifically for what they are— guidelines, but not shackles. It is worth noting that rigid adherence to the original SQUIRE checklist when it was initially published in 2008 resulted in long, even monotonous manuscripts. This was borne out when, as editor-in-chief of *Quality and Safety in Health Care*, I invited three groups of co-authors to test the nascent Guidelines' usefulness for their papers that were undergoing review and revision. The resulting laboriously crafted revisions prompted reviewers to advise—as one voice and unequivocally—that the authors should make selective application of SQUIRE elements in their final published papers [5–7].

This same advice applies today for the author considering use of SQUIRE 2.0 or any other publication guidelines. Make judicious use of the content list to assure a complete report, but above all, never allow its application to be at the cost of crafting an interesting, readable paper. At this point, let us drill down on the specific elements of a typical manuscript in the IMRaD structure.

INTRODUCTION

Your Introduction, at a minimum, addresses a description of your healthcare problem for study, the current knowledge available in the literature about the problem, and the rationale for your unique approach to solving this problem. It should clearly identify the specific aims of the intervention as well as the aims of the paper.

The description of the current problem under study should be brief, but nevertheless an explicit picture of the author's local context that can be recognizable to a reader although that reader is unfamiliar with the author's setting.

The background literature should summarize the current best available knowledge that underlies the initiative. Nevertheless be selective and exercise restraint regarding detail. A critical, selective summary of the relevant available knowledge is much more valuable to the reader than an exhaustive catalogue of every detail in the published literature. This winnowing process is usually a challenge but the author's selectivity provides an enormous service to the reader. Be parsimonious.

Turning to the rationale for the project, it was the consensus of the authors, scholars, and editors that convened for the SQUIRE 2.0 development process [1] that the rationale of a scholarly report can be a difficult and complicated challenge for most authors. Do not underestimate its importance for communicating the broader relevance of your work. First and foremost, it calls for a succinct description of the theory that led to your initiative. The concept of your rationale that underlies the initiative is sufficiently nuanced and important—varying in concept in subtle ways from the classical research hypothesis for initiating laboratory or clinical research—that you will find its many ramifications explored in depth in Chapter 8.

Finally, capture succinctly the specific aim for *this* report—usually the same as the aims of the intervention—in concise, declarative prose. Often this can be achieved in one or two sentences, or a brief bulleted table.

The first time I attended a performance of Puccini's opera *La Bohème,* as I experienced the broad expanse of the performance I gradually became aware that a recurrent and riveting musical theme—the leitmotif—was carrying me from scene to scene. Puccini had crafted this recurring recognizable thread to which everything else was attached. Consider your paper's aim as a leitmotif that reappears in various statements throughout the Methods, Results, Discussion, and Conclusion of the paper. In summary, be parsimonious as you capture your aim, and hang the rest of your paper on this important thread.

METHODS

The Methods section calls for careful presentation of two overarching elements. The first is a description of your improvement intervention together with attention to a vivid picture of your context. The second is a full description of how that improvement process was studied—what measures were selected and how were they analyzed?

Description of the intervention includes a summary of the broad characteristics of the initiative, but it should also include sufficient contextual detail that the reader could decide if it is reasonable to anticipate replicating it in a local setting that might be very different from the author's. The complexity and importance of the context are fully developed in Chapter 7.

Suffice to say here that your description of the physical and organizational attributes of your clinical setting must be broadened to address a wider scope of your context—the role of leadership, culture, external regulations, organizational hierarchy, and other issues that shape the social context for the intervention. A useful way to think about this is to specifically address how your essential contextual elements converged to facilitate your initiative. Stay ever mindful of how your accurate description of these contextual elements might enable the reader to pursue such an initiative in the *reader's* setting.

The second overarching element, the description of the *study of the intervention*, takes your writing task well beyond simply a description of your improvement. The effective use of statistical analysis to establish validity and reproducibility are paramount. Chapter 8 is devoted entirely to this important aspect of your report.

HUMAN SUBJECTS REVIEW

Scholarly journals generally require evidence that you have obtained human subjects review for an improvement initiative before they consider your paper for publication. There are no hard rules about where this information goes in your paper. The authors of SQUIRE 2.0 Guidelines suggest that this information be included at the conclusion of the Methods section in a brief notice described as Ethical Considerations. Some journals prefer it to be included in a specific note that follows the body of your formal paper. The point is not so much where it goes, but rather that it is an essential element that you must pursue early as you contemplate your initiative.

A practical goal, with rare exceptions, is to obtain a waiver from your local research ethics committee (in the United States known as Institutional Review Boards [IRB]), based on the committee's recognition that the initiative is in fact a healthcare improvement initiative, not clinical research *per se*.

RESULTS

Your Results should follow the thread that leads back directly to the aims that were presented in the Introduction and then captured in the Methods sections. It is useful to distinguish explicitly between process outcomes and clinical outcomes in your initiative.

Achievement of measurable change in process outcomes is generally a reportable result, and is often useful to your reader. However, the overall aim of improving patient care relies heavily on reaching a considerably higher bar, improvement in *clinical* outcomes. For example, three reports from Cystic Fibrosis (CF) Care Centers described initiatives that were designed to reduce serious infections [8], improve nutritional status [9] or improve pulmonary function [10], respectively among children with CF. Each paper reported an array of *process* outcomes that were reflected in record keeping, patient and staff educational processes, frequency of visits, and other processes. Of importance, however, these three groups of authors were able to report improvement in the intended *clinical* outcomes. And for even greater emphasis, they compared their respective clinical measures to national trends that were tracked in the CF Network national registry.

There are several ways that your improvement results might differ from those in the usual biomedical clinical report. For example, by their very nature, it is not uncommon for the character and dimensions of improvement results to evolve over time as the implementation process unfolds. Improvement outcomes can have a measure of elasticity that is potentially more complicated than, for example, the binary outcome of a therapeutic trial—the tested therapeutic intervention either works or it does not. To add to your task, these changes inevitably turn around and shape the original context for the intervention—so-called reflexive changes—which should also be captured in the narrative. At the risk of belaboring the point, it is imperative to be mindful of how these contextual changes are likely to be recognizable as relevant to your reader's own clinical and institutional context for continuously improving care [11].

TABLES AND GRAPHS

There are several simple rules for well-designed tables and graphs so that they both amplify and clarify your paper's message. First, put considerable effort into their visual impact. Second, keep tables and graphs as simple as possible. Third, give special attention to the important role that legends play for effectiveness of your tables and graphs. A good rule here is to craft legends so they are sufficiently self-explanatory so that your readers can interpret the graphs and tables without having to refer to the body of the text. On the other hand, refer to your tables and graphs sensibly and logically in the text, and place them strategically in the body of the paper.

DISCUSSION

Your paper's Discussion offers opportunities for you to assure your reader's full grasp of its importance. Nail this down by introducing your Discussion with a succinct summary of your key findings. Craft them in such a way that they lead effectively to the narrative that follows in the Discussion.

In the body of your Discussion, explore in detail where your work fits in the wider literature—the relevance of your results to other similar work, and how it adds to that previous knowledge. This is the place to elaborate further on your paper's meaning and value.

The Limitations section provides an opportunity to go beyond the author's usual *apologia*, which is often presented in anticipation of a reviewer's criticisms. More importantly, here is a place to serve your reader by expanding as well on what you consider the limitations to implementing this work in another setting, particularly that of the reader. Take full advantage here to use the Limitations section for your insights into the difficulties and challenges of replicating it elsewhere.

Finally, your paper's Conclusions offer you one more final shot at a tight summary of the value and meaning of your initiative and its findings. For example, how might they affect patients in other settings and how might your results be useful for other health systems? Enjoy this occasion to celebrate (modestly) your success!

YOUR OBLIGATION TO HELP READERS FIND YOUR PAPER: THE IMPORTANCE OF YOUR TITLE AND ABSTRACT

Remember that many readers will probably encounter your paper only as a title and abstract while scanning a journal's online Table of

Contents. For you to disseminate the most important messages of your paper, this is the place to ensure that such elements are accessible and highlighted effectively.

Put the key message succinctly in the title. Generally avoid the temptation to craft cute, whimsical titles. Such titles are often too esoteric to make your valuable work recognizable. As fun as it is to play with such a title, it rarely snags the intended reader. Adopt such an approach with care. Instead, you can afford to make a title longer, particularly if it adds sufficient description of context and study methodology to be recognizable by your intended reader.

Your paper's abstract requires far more attention and care than its short length might suggest. Since most journals offer abstracts on their websites without financial charge to a passing reader, take advantage of this access to a broad readership. Employ a few simple rules of thumb to enhance your paper's sensibility for the passing reader. Of course, follow your journal's instructions regarding abstract format. Summarize your content in selective, pithy, and interesting prose. Include text headings in the abstract that are taken from the body of the paper to help organize the abstract easily for the reader. Terms that might be unfamiliar to a general reader should be briefly but clearly defined right here in the abstract, and not left to the manuscript's text.

Gil Welch, a colleague at Dartmouth, has suggested crafting an abstract first before writing the text of the paper. Such advice suggests that an early draft abstract can be a useful way for framing the paper before embarking on the text. While Welch's suggestion to employ the abstract as a kind of thumbnail manuscript outline is useful for some authors, I generally urge authors to write the abstract late in the preparation of the paper, particularly as details emerge for the results. Its importance as an online gateway to the text of the paper for interested readers dominates this argument for me. If you prefer to draft it early as a working outline as Welch suggests, revise it frequently in parallel with the text as the final form of the paper emerges.

KEY WORDS AND MESH TERMS

It is valuable for the author to be aware of "searchability" and "findability"—concepts that are generally familiar to bloggers and Internet marketers, but not traditionally considered central to the task of the scholarly author. The author should ask the question, will the reader's use of widely available search software, particularly Google or PubMed, snag this paper? In this regard, work thoughtfully with co-authors to develop appropriate key words and MeSH (Medical Subject Headings) terms. Attention to careful choice of MeSH terms—the National Library of Medicine hierarchy of reference terms—is worth the invested time. This list of reference terms is updated regularly and serves as a common source for the over 5000 biomedical journals in the MedLine/PubMed database.

ON TO YOUR REVISIONS...

Now that you have addressed the important work of developing the elements of your early draft paper, you are positioned to move on to the important work of revision. Your revisions are the careful work that takes your paper from draft to refined submission—what many authors consider the *real* work of writing for publication.

Effective revision is of course the opportunity to step back and explore the big picture of integrating your paper's content and structure. Accordingly, you will find several later chapters devoted to its essential elements. Revision involves closely refining your writing style so that it speaks directly to your reader, integrating the contributions of your co-authors, reflecting again on the critical elements that describe the unique contextual elements of your work, reporting the critical study of your initiative—how and why it worked in your setting—and the detailed refinements of your manuscript that will ultimately prepare it for submission.

DISSEMINATE YOUR MESSAGE: COMMENTARIES, SYSTEMATIC REVIEWS, EDITORIALS, AND LETTERS TO THE EDITOR

In addition to your formal improvement report, consider other formats to amplify your message, for example, letters to the editor, narrative reports, commentaries, and comprehensive systematic reviews. These are but a few of the formats that you will want to consider as you expand the potential impact of your work.

Consider writing a systematic review about your specific research topic. Such a comprehensive review can help to define your place in a community of like-minded scholars. Take advantage of the investment you have made in your background literature review to develop your review. Your improvement report together with your familiarity with this broader literature puts you in a position to serve as an expert. The PRISMA publication guidelines (Preferred Reporting Items for Systematic Reviews and Meta-Analyses) for systematic reviews [12] provide a checklist that most editors expect authors to employ for systematic reviews. Turn to this checklist and stick close to its outline as an effective guide for crafting your review.

Another way to amplify your message is to develop a well-reasoned commentary that derives directly from your improvement findings. Starting with your paper's Conclusions, you might consider elaborating on their significance. What are the messages that capture the logical next directions for answering the open questions that were inevitably raised by your current work? A commentary can also serve to introduce your findings to a broader readership, such as a targeted clinical readership. Consider submitting your commentary to a clinical journal to introduce your work to specialty colleagues who may not routinely be readers of the improvement literature.

Track the evolution of thinking that is initiated by your paper and similar reports. Strategies for scanning the literature include your frequent review of appropriate journal Tables of Contents online, regular searches of the topic by Google and PubMed, and, of course, regular communication with scholars who have similar interests.

If the opportunity presents itself, offer to contribute an editorial on an expanded topic related to your paper, perhaps to the same journal that published your paper. Contact the editor or associate editor who managed the review of your paper with an explicit proposal. Frame your proposal in one paragraph and lead with the defining statement on which your editorial expands. A good rule for both commentaries and editorials is to confine your message to a maximum of four explicit points.

Letters to the Editor are useful vehicles for participation in an ongoing conversation in the literature. If you have a germane perspective on a topic that is raised by a recent journal article, you must be prepared to respond promptly. Many editors expect a letter within 3 weeks of publication of the original article of interest. Adhere closely to the journal's instructions for Letters.

A CODA: HARVESTING REFLECTION, OVERCOMING A DRY WELL, AND FINDING FLOW

Reflection is integral to effective writing—simple, deep reflection. A valuable tool to capture the products of such reflection can be provided by maintaining a personal journal. It will benefit both the improvement under study as well as your writing about it. In this sense, your personal journal serves as your laboratory notebook.

There are of course a myriad of electronic tools that can serve this purpose. Perhaps from years-long habit, I still use a paper format. I have filled dozens of student notebooks over the years. I generally keep my journal nearby and scratch notes when ideas occur—in meetings, at 2 A.M. awakened from sleep, etc. How they emerge is beyond my knowledge of neuroscience, but they come at odd times. I once asked a carpenter friend who lives in the same small town as I, if he would provide me his most creative ideas about how to provide a more effective workspace and study for writing. I agreed to compensate him for his drawings. His response, "You know sometimes my best ideas come when I'm just driving around from job to job in my truck." I readily agreed that was compensable time—as it turned out, some of the most valuable.

Additions to your journal over the course of an improvement initiative provide a valuable source for rich material—insights into what actually happened as it unfolded. These substantive qualitative data provide material for retrospective analysis of the complex social processes that are woven into your initiative. Allow some time and distance to unfold for you to analyze these data critically. We will return to their utility in Chapter 8 where we explore the process of ex post analysis and theory development.

WHEN THE WELL SEEMS DRY

Sometimes nothing seems to appear on the page or screen. How do you get started with a manuscript when nothing is forthcoming? How can you write when the well seems dry? Blocked.

One colleague at Dartmouth says when this happens, she reads. Anything. I have tried it and it works for me too. Reading fiction oddly has served as well as the professional journal article that is sitting on my desk. Do not shy away from trying your own experiments in this regard. If your writing is blocked, read.

Other suggestions from Dartmouth trainees and faculty for dislodging what many call writer's block included the following. "Sometimes (*rarely*) there's some kind of muse at work, but when it's not there, often I just have to power forward with a 'forced march' draft—writing anything just to get started!" "The more frequently I write, the easier it is to get started the next time. Even if it's just 15 minutes at a time." "I use my journal—bedside, front seat of my car, wherever. It provides kernels to pick up when I next sit down to write."

We concluded that several things can serve to facilitate keeping the writing process on track—principally strategies to develop continuity in your writing. One is to finish each writing session with a well-defined task to begin next time. A short note to oneself with the unfinished task serves this purpose. Many reported that writing momentum could be nudged by something as simple as a regular time for uninterrupted scholarly writing. Providing enough time for writing is also required. We will explore further how many successful authors wedge their writing into busy professional and personal lives in Chapter 6.

FINDING FLOW

Occasionally a surprising reward occurs—a draft just seems to flow onto the page. While writing often involves difficult, slogging work, one is occasionally rewarded by arriving at what some call a state of "flow." This is the moment when the process turns from labor to something else—something easy and natural. The writing process seems simply to fully take over one's consciousness. One cannot force the process since it unfolds in its own good time. It creates its own momentum. Flow—or whatever you may call this—does not often occur, but when it does, you will find that such a level of concentration becomes its own reward.

Now, it is onto a dive into the several elements that can contribute further to your writing success, starting in the next chapter with finding your intended reader and developing an effective writing style.

REFERENCES

1. Ogrinc G, Davies L, Goodman D, Batalden P, Davidoff F, Stevens D. SQUIRE 2.0 (Standards for QUality Improvement Excellence): Revised publication guidelines from a detailed consensus process. *BMJ Qual Saf*. Published online first doi:10.1136/bmjqs-2015-004411. Published simultaneously in: *Am Journal of Medical Quality; Canadian Journal of Diabetes; Joint Commission Journal on Quality and Patient Safety; Journal of Nursing Care Quality; American Journal of Critical Care; The Permanente Journal; Evidence: Open access journal of GIMBE Foundation for Evidence Based Health Care; Medwave – Chile. Online; Journal of the American College of Surgeons; and Journal of Surgical Research.*

2. Pinnock H, Barwick M, Carpenter CR, et al. Standards for reporting implementation Studies. *BMJ* 2017;356:i6795 doi:101136/bmj.i6795.

3. Goodman D, Ogrinc G, Davies L, et al. Explanation and elaboration of the SQUIRE 2.0 (Standards for QUality Improvement Excellence) Guidelines, V. 2.0: Examples of SQUIRE elements in the healthcare improvement literature. *BMJ Qual Saf*: Published online first doi:10.1136/ bmjqs-2015-004480.

4. Holzmueller CG, Pronovost PJ. Organising a manuscript reporting quality improvement or patient safety research. *BMJ Qual Saf* 2013;22:777–785.

5. Bechtold ML, Scott S, Nelson K, Cox KR, Dellsperger KC, Hall LW. Educational quality improvement report: Outcomes from a revised morbidity and mortality format that emphasized patient safety. *Qual Saf Health Care* 2007;16:422–427.

6. Kirsh SR, Aron DC. Integrating the chronic-care model and the ACGME competencies: Using shared medical appointments to focus on systems-based practice. *Qual Saf Health Care* 2008;17:15–19.

7. Hoffman KG, Brown RMA, Gay JW, Headrick LA. How an educational improvement project improved the summative evaluation of medical students. *Qual Saf Health Care* 2009;18:283–287.

8. Savant AP, O'Malley C, Bichl S, McColley SA. Improved patient safety through reduced airway infection rates in a pediatric cystic fibrosis program after a quality improvement effort to enhance infection prevention and control measure. *BMJ Qual Saf* 2014;23:i73–i80.

9. Savant AP, Britton LC, Petren K, McColley SA, Gutierrez HH. Sustained improvement in nutritional outcomes at two pediatric cystic fibrosis centers after quality improvement collaboratives. *BMJ Qual Saf* 2014;23:i81–i89.

10. Zanni RL, Sembrano EU, Du DT, Marra B, Bantang R. The impact of re-education of airway clearance techniques (REACT) on adherence and pulmonary function in patients with cystic fibrosis. *BMJ Qual Saf* 2014;23:i50–i55.

11. Stevens DP, Shojania KG. Tell me about the context, and more. *BMJ Qual Saf* 2011;20:557–559.

12. Moher D, Liberati A, Tetzlaff J, Altman DG, The PRISMA Group. Preferred Reporting Items for Systematic Reviews and Meta-Analyses: The PRISMA Statement. *PLoS Med.* 2009;6(7):e1000097. PMID: 19621072.

CHAPTER 3
Develop a writing style that focuses on your reader

FOCUS ON YOUR READER

Write for your reader. While this is good advice for all authors, such mindfulness is particularly central to writing to improve healthcare. Of fundamental importance here is the fact that your reader ultimately is integral to achieving the essential aim of your healthcare improvement writing—translating your improvement work into better patient care.

Direct communication with your reader involves two essential elements. The first element is your deep *knowledge* of your reader. How can you possibly know your reader, this stranger who scans a Table of Contents and decides to read your paper? How might you address this transcendent question?

An equally important second element to achieving this connection with your reader is an accessible, sensible writing style. We will pursue both these elements in detail.

IDENTIFYING YOUR READER

A concerted focus on the reader is probably more familiar to authors and readers of serious fiction than aspirants to scholarly scientific writing. I gained a better understanding for this by listening carefully to my friend and colleague, Rita Charon, who is a professor of medicine and founder of the Program in Narrative Medicine at

Columbia University in New York City. This innovative author, physician, and Henry James scholar has explored her deep insights into the unique author-reader relationship in her groundbreaking book, *Narrative Medicine* [1].

The author–reader connection in fiction may seem a long way from your relationship with your healthcare improvement reader. Or is it? Charon has probed this uniquely existential process that joins the writer and the reader—one human with another. She has referred to this as "a communion of sorts," this relationship that exists between a teller and listener, and—particularly relevant to our purposes here—between author and reader [1].

Does this concept of communion, with all its suggestion of empathy, closeness, and—dare I say, intimacy—really have anything to do with your writing to improve healthcare? Absolutely. An unobstructed path to your reader is a substantial part of your reader's gaining a grasp of the complex sociologic and psychological elements that can serve to adapt your work to your reader's setting. There are several pragmatic steps that will start you on this process.

SIMPLE STRATEGIES THAT CAN SMOOTH THE PATH TO YOUR READER

A starting point is simply to reflect upfront on this question: who is your reader? Literally visualize your reader and how he or she is likely to find your message to be valuable for local healthcare improvement. This will require explicit attention to how you use language to frame your case for improvement.

The journalist, Verlyn Klinkenborg, brings another perspective to this communion. He urges the author to flip this question about your reader—to think in terms of who *you* are to your *reader* [2]. How does your world and that of your reader overlap? On reflection, this can lead readily to several straightforward decisions in your early drafts.

For one thing, it calls for care that certain words do not get in the way of useful communication. For example, think critically about two "naming" decisions—on the surface two seemingly simple definitions. First, how do you label the human subjects in your initiative? Secondly, how do you name your participants' professional work? Be sure this naming harmonizes with how *you* and your *reader* perceive your roles in healthcare.

How might your reader characterize his or her professional identity? Respect this view by being as specific as possible as you name a critical care physician or nurse, endocrinologist, surgeon or primary care clinician. Who is providing that care, for example, "doctors," "nurses," "clinicians," "healthcare workers," or "providers"? Here, the greatest specificity carries the day. Similarly, the narrative will have a slightly different focus if the answer to this question is "hospital CEO," "nursing leader," or "practice manager." The rationale for getting this right is your imperative to connect as efficiently and simply with your reader—the unseen colleague who is likely to provide the leverage for advancing healthcare improvement based on reading about your initiative.

This leads to a second similar naming decision—how do you label the human subjects in your initiative. Be ever mindful of the variety of such definitions and how they vary across segments of the professional community. They can be freighted with a variety of nuanced albeit unintentional messages for different readers. The purpose again here is to be as accessible to your reader as possible, to avoid the risk of creating the slightest turn-off with inadvertently dissonant jargon. For example, are the initiative's subjects "patients" or "clients"? Is the report about the "healthcare industry," "healthcare systems" or maybe simply a "hospital"? Such word choices can either facilitate the acceptance of an important message, or do the opposite—subtly but ever so surely impede your successful communication. Take the time to reach early consensus on these simple decisions with your co-authors and be consistent throughout your manuscript.

JUST HOW MANY READERS WILL YOUR PAPER FIND?

Professional musicians have told me that they perform with the same intensity and commitment for as many or as few listeners that show up to hear their performance. The point here is that the goal for a serious performer is not the size of the crowd; it is to play for those few or many listeners who can truly hear and be moved by the performance.

Not to be the skunk in the garden party, but reflect for a moment on just how many readers might realistically read your paper after its publication in a scholarly journal. While a journal's formal circulation may number in the thousands, can you actually assume that will be the number of readers who read your paper online or in print? On the other hand, it is your obligation to write for that specific cohort of *your* readers as precisely as possible, regardless of the actual number. If you and your co-authors have done your work well to identify that cohort, the number will be less important than the process whereby your work ultimately leads to the improvement of their patients' care and their healthcare systems.

WORK TO ACHIEVE AN EFFECTIVE WRITING STYLE

Much of this book up to this point has addressed the "what"—the content of your scholarly healthcare improvement report. You have an additional obligation—the difficult work of the "how" of writing—the achievement of an accessible, interesting writing style. Entire manuals have been devoted to writing style—how the author uses words effectively to craft a successful article. Three titles that offer guidance to achieving an effective writing style in the scientific fields include *AMA Manual of Style. A Guide for Authors and Editors* [3], *Writing Science in Plain English* [4], and *The Craft of Scientific Communication* [5]. They offer helpful, interesting, and engaging advice on crafting readable, publishable, accessible biomedical science reports. Their scope is broad, but they do not speak directly to the effective style that is imperative for you as a healthcare improvement author.

At stake here is your success in taking hold of the reader's attention, maintaining interest and thereby inviting a reader to see his or her path to implementing your improvement innovation. A generous, readable, interesting, and easy prose is a large part of this task. This is about both your style and the writing craft that will lead to that style. Consider at least 4 elements for such a writing style: clarity, parsimony, color, and rhythm.

ELEMENTS OF AN EFFECTIVE STYLE: CLARITY

Klinkenborg insists that style *per se* may not actually be the issue. He insists the important point here is *clarity* [2]. Working at your writing *craft* to cultivate simple sentences, and plain prose is an important strategy for achieving this clarity. Comb through your draft for the long sentences, convoluted syntax, repeating lists—*this* list is endless. Search for and eliminate overused—and generally meaningless words—like "very" or "significant" (do you mean "substantial"?). Assure that your message comes through with simple power and moment.

Healthcare professionals are renowned for their jargon that historically served to define the separation between professional and lay communities. Not so in this era. The possibility for jargon creeping into your prose is even greater when you add the additional lexicon of healthcare improvement science to all the catalogues that we use as doctors, nurses, and administrators. Go on a mission to purge your draft of every trace of jargon. Replace it with useful, meaningful prose.

ELEMENTS OF AN EFFECTIVE STYLE: PARSIMONY

As a healthcare improvement author, you have much to say, but explore carefully how parsimony will facilitate your message. Parsimony—close relative of clarity—is difficult work. The seventeenth century French physicist and theologian, Blaise Pascal, made clear just how difficult when he wrote the often-paraphrased comment, "I would have written a shorter letter, but I didn't have the time." Quaker guidance regarding meeting utterances is probably good advice here. "Keep close to the root" to "avoid all vain and distracting ornamentation."

The award-winning actor Mark Rylance alluded to parsimony when he discussed his performance as Thomas Cromwell in the BBC presentation of Hilary Mantel's *Wolf Hall*. He spoke in his usual understated (and parsimonious) style during a WBUR Boston Public Radio interview on January 14, 2016. Rylance described what he discovered of Cromwell's thoughts and reasoning in the gift of Mantel's prose and how it smoothed the path to his performance—one or two carefully chosen words that captured the gist of several pages of Mantel's eloquent prose [6].

Similar advice that applies to your writer's craft is Mark Twain's harsh counsel, "You have to be willing to kill your firstborn." Now *that* puts this in pretty startling terms! When I am revising, painfully pruning, and pruning some more, Twain's words frequently come to mind.

One way I have been able to ease the pain of such literary filicide is to create a file for each manuscript labeled "Cutting Room Floor." I cut and paste deletions to this file. I have been able more readily to cast them aside in a place where they are not fully sacrificed. At late stages of preparation of a paper, I will return to scan this file, often over a dozen pages long, to see if there were any brilliance there that should be rescued. Reassuringly enough, I rarely salvage much for the manuscript.

The author-aviator Saint-Exupery admonished, "You're not finished when there's nothing more to add. You're finished when there's nothing more to cut." I fantasize Saint-Exupery peering over my shoulder (with Twain next to the other shoulder, if you can picture this) as I reach the late revisions of a manuscript.

ELEMENTS OF AN EFFECTIVE STYLE: COLOR AND RHYTHM

Now comes Virginia Woolf, who is said to have written, "Style is a very simple matter: it is all rhythm." What do you imagine she was talking about?

One afternoon a number of years ago, I attended a master class at the Cleveland Institute of Music offered by the remarkable Russian cellist, Mstislav Rostropovich. Master classes are assembled to offer students the opportunity to experience a few precious minutes coaching with a visiting master. A student is chosen to perform a brief movement or passage from a recognizable classical work, and the teacher offers guidance, often performing exemplary passages as a way to reflect style and artistry.

A master class experience can be riveting—some would say grueling—for the student who is usually chosen for her expertise and resilience. On this occasion, the student was a masters degree student in her early twenties. As she began to play her cello—I recall it was a prelude from a Bach cello suite—Rostropovich graciously leaned back and listened. But it was not long before the unfortunate student's rather perfunctory performance seemed to disturb his demeanor. Finally, unable to continue, he interrupted (a familiar convention for a master class) and said simply, "You seem to play everything mezzo-forte. You are what I would call an accomplished mezzo-fortist!"

Mezzo-forte may seem easier to grasp as a musical concept; but as an aspiring author, reflect on how you might effectively develop color and rhythm for your prose. There are approaches to this that are probably as technical as learning the cello fingering for the Bach Prelude. For example, how might individual word choice accomplish this? Then, examine carefully the pace and intensity of a particular phrase, sentence, or paragraph. Consider also such techniques as varying the length of sentences, or the careful choice of words that can surprise. Avoid the temptation to reach for complicated phrases, when simple ones will serve.

Focus—but not too self-consciously—on color and rhythm. I find it is a constant technical challenge when working toward an appealing and interesting style.

STARE AT SOMETHING UNTIL YOU SEE IT: AN EXERCISE IN CLOSE READING

So for Klinkenborg, style is clarity, for Pascal, parsimony, and for Woolf, rhythm. It is of course all these elements and more. How then might you think productively about developing your own effective improvement writing style?

"Stare at something until you see it." Attributed to the French sculptor, Auguste Rodin, this advice serves the aspiring writer well. Practice the habit of awareness of the contribution that each new article that you read can make to your own writing. Charon calls this process simply "close reading." She develops an explicit approach to close reading in her classes and you will find an extended explanation in *Narrative Medicine* [1]. Her description advances five elements for consideration—*frame, form, time, plot, and desire*. On reflection, these are elements that can be found in just about anything from fiction to a patient's clinical record [1]. How might you apply these terms to healthcare improvement reports? How indeed? I urge you to try adapting these 5 elements to an exercise in close reading. Start by selecting the most recent article that you found useful for your own improvement work and use these elements as organizing concepts. You need not force a fit here. Keep it simple.

FIND YOUR OWN EXAMPLES OF GOOD WRITING

We experimented with several other approaches to close reading with the Dartmouth residents and faculty in our writing collaborative. Every year we would spend at least one full session with the aim of developing a list of exceptional healthcare improvement authors (see Appendix).

We initiated the exercise by asking each participant to reflect on examples of what he or she considered interesting, memorable scholarly writing. We would then explore what characteristics led to inclusion in such a list. The list of characteristics started with an author's readability. Pressed to define this more clearly, there was agreement that such a writing style was invariably marked by a succinct narrative, sometimes effective humor, and always simple, declarative prose.

Table 3.1 summarizes a short list of authors that emerged from the discussion. The list includes the innovative UK sociologist, Mary Dixon-Woods, British primary care scholar, Trish Greenhalgh, the U.S. professor of medicine and editor, Bob Wachter, the American

Table 3.1 A limited list of authors that a group of Dartmouth resident trainees and their faculty selected as examples of writing worthy of study

Author	Reasons for inclusion	Representative references
Mary Dixon-Woods	Innovative sociologist's perspective presented in explicit, persuasive, direct prose	Dixon-Woods M et al. What counts? An ethnographic study of infection data reported to a safety program. *Milbank Quarterly* 2012; 90:548–591.
Trisha Greenhalgh	Creative perspective presented with humor and irony	Greenhalgh T et al. Why national health programs need dead philosophers. Wittgensteinian reflections on policymakers' reluctance to learn from history. *Milbank Quarterly* 2011; 89:533–563.
Robert Wachter	A prolific writer and clear thinker with an ever-fresh perspective on health systems	Wachter RM. Observation status for hospitalized patients. A maddening policy begging for revision. *JAMA Int Med* 2013;173: 1999–2000.

(Continued)

Table 3.1 (*Continued*) A limited list of authors that a group of Dartmouth resident trainees and their faculty selected as examples of writing worthy of study

Author	Reasons for inclusion	Representative references
Frank Davidoff	A senior editor's fresh look at unfamiliar topics	Davidoff F. Heterogeneity is not always noise. Lessons from improvement. *JAMA* 2009; 302:2580–2586.
Lisa Rubenstein	A framer of probing questions that move the field to new ground	Rubenstein L, Khodyakov D, Hempel S, Danz M, Salem-Schatz S, Foy R, O'Neil S, Dalal S, Shekelle P. How can we recognize continuous quality improvement? *Int J Qual Health Care* 2014; 26:6–15.
Atul Gawande	A lucid writer who frames complex issues for health professionals and the non-expert lay reader	Gawande A. Postscript: Oliver Sacks. *The New Yorker*. September 14, 2015 Issue.
Harlan Krumholz	An innovative researcher and prolific writer for diverse communities	Krumholz HM. Perspective. Post-hospital syndrome— An acquired, transient condition of generalized risk. *N Engl J Med* 2013;368:100–102.

endocrinologist, Frank Davidoff, the creative RAND scholar, Lisa Rubenstein, the Harvard surgeon, Atul Gawande, and the Yale cardiologist and health services scholar, Harlan Krumholz. These are provided here as examples. We quickly became aware that such a list inevitably omits writers that others would insist are exemplary.

Over time I have developed a habit of reading anything I encounter by these authors. Always time well spent, it serves many purposes including discovery of exceptional writing, stimulating fresh ideas, and simple reading enjoyment. Reflect on your own favorite authors. What are your criteria for inclusion? Or read again several of the references that you find in the Table and come to your own conclusions. Develop your own list as you probe other authors' style for clues that might inform your own writing.

It should be clear by now that there are several strategies for approaching close reading from your unique writer's perspective. Develop your own systematic strategies that can add the greatest contribution to your own writing craft. You might start with a search for examples of clarity, parsimony, color, and rhythm. For example, after reading the Introduction, how did the author eliminate any question of why this initiative was undertaken? How does this author establish a clear aim that builds expectations for the rest of the narrative? What is the craft that extends this thread easily through the Methods to the Results? As you begin to read the Discussion, how has this author clearly summarized her sense of the meaning of the findings? Is there clarity in the relation of these results to the larger healthcare environment? Is the prose parsimonious? Find your own examples of economical phrasing and simple syntax. Where are examples of careful nuance that add color? Does the pace add to a reader's interest—perhaps something as simple as variation in sentence length?

EMPLOY YOUR OWN STRATEGIES FOR READING TO BE A BETTER WRITER

Bottom line: when you have finished reading, do you have the sense that this author spoke directly to you? Were there elements of empathy that spoke to your role as a reader who seeks to improve healthcare?

It is as simple as this. Be systematic in your reading to be a better author.

REFERENCES

1. Charon R. (2006). *Narrative Medicine. Honoring the Stories of Illness*, pp. 52–53 and 114–127. New York, NY: Oxford University Press.
2. Klinkenborg V. (2012). *Several Short Sentences About Writing*, p. 204. New York, NY: Alfred A. Knopf.
3. JAMA editors and staff. (2007). *AMA Manual of Style. A Guide for Authors and Editors*, 10th ed. New York, NY: Oxford University Press.
4. Greene AE. (2013). *Writing Science in Plain English*. Chicago, IL: University of Chicago Press.
5. Harmon JE, Gross AG. (2010). *The Craft of Scientific Communication*. Chicago, IL: University of Chicago Press.
6. http://www.wbur.org/radioboston/2016/01/14/fish-rylance-kampen. Accessed September 2, 2017.

CHAPTER 4
Writing efficiently and effectively with co-authors

"IF YOU CAN'T DESCRIBE WHAT YOU'RE DOING AS A PROCESS, YOU DON'T KNOW WHAT YOU'RE DOING."

W. Edwards Deming defined in this simple, but emphatic admonition a perspective that we ignore at our peril as we contemplate our work with co-authors. Truth be told, however, the working partnership with co-authors is often an ad hoc series of processes at best—often burdened with elements of waste and delay.

Each manuscript brings a new set of social and professional dynamics among co-authors, even if you have worked together as colleagues on previous professional activities. As your paper progresses from revision to revision, the work associated with each revision will invariably take on a course of its own. The pace and direction of this course is difficult to anticipate at the outset. However, a few general rules will help anticipate its trajectory and can yield a substantial measure of efficiency. I urge you to invest the time and effort at reaching consensus on this process at an early meeting of your co-authors.

The complex interactions with your co-authors are generally unique for your specific improvement initiative and manuscript. On the other hand, there are process-driven opportunities that are common to every co-author interaction—generalizable strategies that can allow you to take advantage of familiar improvement techniques. They will be recognizable to most healthcare improvement professionals and inevitably can lead to greater efficiency and effectiveness.

Frame your co-author collaboration so that it is a successful process that builds on the careful work that constituted your early drafts. At its best, it will be highly creative and productive. The dominant aim is a relentless focus on developing a successful paper for journal submission. On the other hand, left to a random process, effective revision can be burdened with unanticipated inefficiency and waste. Because of the emotional and professional investments that each co-author brings to the work, I urge you to hew to Demming's advice, and do the early work to frame your work with your co-authors as an effective, definable process. These process elements are readily found at the various milestones in the continuum of a manuscript's development from first draft to submitted manuscript and published paper.

USING IMPROVEMENT METHODOLOGY TO ENHANCE WRITING PRODUCTIVITY

Process maps, fishbone diagrams, run charts, and small tests of change that employ Plan-Do-Study-Act cycles in your writing processes are all examples of improvement methodology that can contribute to your success together as co-authors. Neuhauser et al. suggested employing fishbone diagrams to capture reasons for loss of momentum—process elements that go straight at barriers no matter how seemingly mundane [1]. You will likely recognize causes that they found in categories such as *personal* ("diddling around, fatigue"); *resources* ("computer availability, adapter plugs [!], need references data"), *environment* ("plane too crowded, 70+ hour workweek, morning after late night, morning meetings"), and *other demands* ("time on calendar, travel, interruptions, preparation for teaching"). Run charts can track the time required for a revision of a particular section, the time that is effectively committed to writing each day, or daily productivity as measured simply by the number of words that are produced each day. This investment in process analysis can provide useful insights. Consider crafting a fishbone diagram or process design for your own personal writing as well as that of your work with your co-authors.

However, there is still more to the complex collaborative work with co-authors. It is worth taking a deeper dive into the several layers that will support its success. There is a payoff here.

THE NOT SO OBVIOUS IMPEDIMENTS

While scholarly writing starts in private, authors frequently find the act of moving a preliminary draft to the first review by another reader to be a startling encounter—filled with the risk, even terror, of exposing one's inner thoughts to the glare of another's view.

This subtle impediment does not inevitably accompany writing with colleagues, but take a moment to acknowledge the emotional freight that can potentially accompany sharing early writing products with colleagues. Most professionals generally assume these—often unconscious—issues were resolved somewhere in early school days. At the risk of belaboring this point, successful writing with colleagues can be accelerated simply by early acknowledgement of the trepidation that co-authors may experience when they share an early draft with colleagues.

A central aspect of this work together with your co-authors is that it interweaves two essential roles that co-authors bring to the work together—that of both author and reviewer. Reflecting on this dualism can become the foundation for shared pedagogy and improvement for all your co-authors. Peer review itself is actually an improvement process and sufficiently complex for the success of your paper; you will find it explored in detail in the next chapter.

IDENTIFYING APPROPRIATE CO-AUTHORS

There are decisions that must be addressed early and explicitly if the path for your paper from first draft to published paper is to avoid unanticipated disruptions. Obvious as it may seem as a first decision, identify the appropriate co-authors for your manuscript as early as possible—a decision that is not always as straightforward as it might seem.

There are acknowledged conventions that apply and can be helpful for these decisions. All co-authors should merit inclusion by their meaningful contribution to the paper and the work it reports. It is useful to identify and maintain clarity about each one's specific contribution. The International Committee of Medical Journal Editors (ICMJE) provides widely acknowledged guidelines for inclusion criteria for co-authors [2]. Journals increasingly require that you attest to specific adherence to these guidelines.

Identification of the first and last authors generally requires special attention. Consensus should be established early regarding who will be the principal (first) author, presumably you. As straightforward as this may seem, it should be established unequivocally early to avoid unexpressed assumptions about this among colleagues.

The first author serves in a chief executive role, and journals identify the first author as the point of contact and coordinator of the editing and revision process. The paper is inevitably drafted in the writing style of the first author, but there can be stylistic pressures raised by edits from co-authors. Nevertheless, for the writing process to work efficiently, co-authors should defer whenever possible to the first author's direction.

The last name in the list of authors is frequently the most senior scholar—for example, a department chair or section chief. Just like all other co-authors, his or her inclusion should meet ICMJE criteria for contributions to the project and paper, and not be determined by position in the institutional hierarchy. On occasion, this issue can require highly sophisticated navigation of treacherous academic political shoals. Given the diversity and complexity of institutional cultures, there is unfortunately little generalizable, useful advice that I can offer here except for the utility of diplomatically citing ICMJE chapter and verse.

WORKING TOGETHER AS A HIGH PERFORMANCE MICROSYSTEM

The variability that is found among different kinds of organizational small groups has been studied and has relevance here. Arrow and colleagues describe recurring common themes that characterize small groups as complex systems [3]. In this vein, a useful strategy for you and your co-authors to consider is to anchor your work together in principles that have been described for high-performance microsystems [4].

The ethnographic research that has characterized The High Performance Clinical Microsystem has focused specifically on the work of clinical units and how they effectively worked together for efficient, safe patient care [4]. These same principles can be adapted usefully to the processes of co-authors' work together. The following overarching microsystem principles are reframed to apply to your work together as co-authors.

1. The co-author team is a micro-organization with a set of defined aims, for example, efficient production of a manuscript that will serve patients and health systems.
2. As such it relies on shared and linked information processes that interact with the broader environment such as local library resources and, more broadly, Internet access to the relevant literature.
3. In a practical sense, it meets certain defined needs of co-authors, for example, their shared professional stakes in a successfully published manuscript.
4. The writing work of co-authors is imbedded in a complex adaptive system—their larger healthcare and/or academic organization. Specifically, for example, co-authors each have a professional and personal life that must accommodate the work of the paper's development.

Now take each of these overarching principles to a more pragmatic level. Toward this end, the Dartmouth LPMR trainees and faculty developed a list of generalizable expectations for co-authors' work together (also see Appendix).

Consensus on these expectations at an early face-to-face meeting of co-authors can be well worth the investment. It will serve to avoid wasteful false starts early on, and misunderstandings later as writing together unfolds.

The LPMR trainees and faculty developed consensus around a list that I have modified and revised in the following nine pragmatic interpersonal elements. Many of these elements will seem obvious to you. Nevertheless, you will discover that your work as an effective microsystem will benefit from their acknowledgement by all participants.

1. Agree to demonstrate respect for each other but also agree to reflect brutal honesty.
2. At a foundational level, all co-authors should conscientiously practice giving and receiving effective feedback for each serial revision.

In this regard, everyone should agree to the general rule of holding one's own products lightly while entertaining others' proposed options.

3. Clearly acknowledge each person's strengths and weaknesses. Consider assigning appropriate sections to the most expert co-author, such as the statistician, qualitative scholar, or administrative expert, so that the paper will reflect the strengths of each.

4. Commit to maintaining momentum in the writing process. This will be served by agreeing upon a structure and explicit timeline for the drafting work. Establish who crafts the first draft—presumably the first author. Agree to a process for co-authors' response with firm internal draft-to-draft deadlines, returning revisions in timely fashion for collation by the first author.

5. Respect time, space, and individual professional boundaries, but the paper must take high priority in the work of all so that momentum is maintained. Simple as this commitment may seem, a practical consideration for timely completion of writing tasks requires that all participants provide access via their direct email address and telephone number.

6. Assure that the same word-processing technology is available to all. Keep it simple. This is not the time for testing a new technology, or one that has been used by a minority of the co-authors. There are several software applications for shared access to revisions such as those available via Google or Drop Box. All must be willing to use such an application if it is to facilitate rather than complicate the process. Given the variability of e-skills, many co-author teams still decide to default to a work process that relies on email attachments of Track-Change revisions.

7. Be clear about how key decisions will be made if there are differences of opinion. Examples can include such features as aim, key messages, intended target readership, and journal choice. Arbitrary decisions may be necessary if and when there is poor consensus among the majority. This generally falls to you as first author, and all must agree that there will be such an adjudication process in the rare event that there is deadlock. Agreement in advance to such a firm rule will go far to head off potential permanent fracture of personal and professional relationships.

8. Attend early to a set of "First Tasks" that will pull together the work of your co-author team around a set of explicit decisions.

9. As the paper reaches late draft stages, designate colleagues who practice being an outsider. An additional and useful strategy for bringing fresh eyes to the work is to find a hypercritical colleague who is willing to play this role. We will learn more about that later.

"FIRST TASKS" FOR YOUR WORK TOGETHER ON THE MANUSCRIPT AT HAND

Now turn to consideration of two "first tasks:" identifying co-authors' explicit stakes in this project, and unequivocal clarity about the paper's aim. These decisions will require recurring, regular attention by you and your co-authors. They are emphasized here because of their importance and priority.

Begin by identifying your co-authors' shared investments in the project, explicitly identifying each participant's stake in the project. For example, a pragmatic professional career issue for most co-authors will be meeting expectations for departmental scholarly productivity goals—important for career retention and promotion. While it may be assumed that these are shared investments, it is valuable to identify them along with other co-author stakes early in the writing project. It is valuable to call out a shared aim for most co-authors—the dissemination of a successful initiative for your eventual readers to adopt for the benefit of patients and health systems.

Another "first task" is to reach agreement on the aim for *this* paper at the outset of work together, and maintain focus on the aim as revisions evolve. "What? I thought the initiative had a clear aim when we embarked on the project." While establishing the aim was part of your original initiative as reflected in your first draft, this is an element that requires consensus by your entire co-author group as you set about work together. Furthermore, while the aim(s) might seem self-evident to you as principal author, if there is disagreement among co-authors, it will surface in many ways along the way—false starts at revisions that are based on misaligned assumptions or misunderstandings about desired publication outcomes.

How might the aim for the paper diverge from that of the initiative? While it will generally harmonize with the initiative's aim, the paper may have a second emphasis on presenting particular aspects of the work. Examples can include detailed exploration of a particular methodology, a surprising aspect of a subset of results, or a separate deep dive into policy or cost implications of the initiative. Such a discussion might lead to a broader co-authors' publication strategy for the initiative.

SEEK INFORMAL CRITICAL READS BY COLLEAGUES

A final step before submission of your paper to an editor's sharp eye is to ask one or more colleagues who are not co-authors to give the manuscript a critical read. Choose colleagues that share professional interests with your anticipated reader. This test by a colleague is a considerable gift before releasing your careful work to the wider arc of a journal's editorial and review processes. Consider asking him or her to read your paper using Wager and Godley's three reviewers' questions: Do I understand it? Do I believe it? Do I Care? [5].

This is a reasonable place to examine in depth the full contribution of *peer review* to your paper's success. Peer review is itself an improvement process that contains important elements for your paper to reach its full potential.

REFERENCES

1. Neuhauser D, McEachern E, Zyzanski S, Flocke S, Williams RL. Continuous quality improvement and the process of writing for academic publications. *Qual Manag Health Care* 2000;8:65–73.
2. International Committee of Medical Journal Editors. *Defining the Role of Authors and Contributors*. http://www.icmje.org/recommendations/browse/roles-and-responsibilities/defining-the-role-of-authors-and-contributors.html. Accessed July 13, 2016.
3. Arrow H, McGrath JE, Berdahl JL. (2000). *Small Groups as Complex Systems. Formation, Coordination, Development and Adaptation*. Thousand Oaks, CA: Sage Publications.
4. Nelson EC, Batalden PB, Huber TP, et al. Microsystems in healthcare: Part 1. Learning from high-performing frontline clinical units. *Joint Comm J Qual and Safety*;28:472–493.
5. Wager E, Godlee F, Jefferson T. (2002). *How to Survive Peer Review*. London: BMJ Books.

CHAPTER 5
Harness the full potential of peer review for your writing success

PEER REVIEW AND ITS CONTRIBUTION TO YOUR WRITING

Your manuscript progresses along a continuum that starts with your first draft and ultimately leads to your successful publication in a journal. That continuum is marked by interfaces between you and colleagues who provide critical reviews to your paper's continuous improvement, thereby contributing substantially to your writing success at every stage—colleagues, co-authors, editors, and reviewers. Finally, it can be said that the reader who discovers your published paper will be your reviewer of greatest importance.

Writing—transferring thoughts from your brain to a screen or page—is a complex and challenging undertaking. Moreover, drafting your paper is a very private and challenging activity, but when you bring on this complex interaction between you as an author and colleagues, co-authors, editors, and journal reviewers, both opportunities and challenges emerge. This interaction repeats again and again, albeit in different forms as your draft gains ever-wider circulation among such reviewers. A relatively informal review by a colleague of your earliest, loosely assembled first draft provides perspectives that serve your writing quite differently from the formal process that constitutes a formal review at the request of a journal editor. They all contribute to this process that helps you accomplish your ultimate aim—an accessible, sensible paper for a community of journal readers.

While a wide range of reviewers will provide different contributions as your manuscript develops, their contributions share many of the same principles. Nevertheless, these interactions between you and your reviewers take place on a scholarly foundation that is anchored on a startling fact. There is little evidence from hundreds of studies to explain either how peer review works or even how to improve the peer review process itself. That is probably a good place to start.

PEER REVIEW AS AN IMPROVEMENT PROCESS

How in the world does peer review work—in all its complexity? When you reflect on this process, you find that a successfully published paper is invariably a better paper, and considerably different from the paper that you originally conceived and drafted. The learning theory that underlies peer review aligns best with Kolb's theory of adult experiential learning [1], an elegantly simple theory that describes the cyclical pattern whereby adults generally learn. The cycle starts first with the learner's experience. He or she observes and reflects on this experience. Such reflection is followed by formulation of abstract concepts that are based on that reflection. Finally, the learner tests those concepts in new experiences. Does this look like something else that might be familiar to you as a healthcare improvement professional? There is much about Kolb's theory that is in harmony with learning and improvement processes associated with Plan-Do-Study-Act cycles of classical process improvement.

What is the evidence for the contribution of peer review in scientific publication? For centuries peer review has been a staple of scholarly publication, as it has been for other elements of scientific affairs—for example, evaluation for the award of grants or academic promotion.

Many scholars have studied this process in efforts to develop the evidence for peer review's specific role in scientific publication. Unfortunately, systematic reviews of available studies have provided inconsistent evidence at best. To be sure, studies appear to demonstrate a positive contribution for such elements as training referees, the utility of statistical checklists, or the value of concealing reviewer and author identities. Probably the most encouraging outcome of these analyses is the generally consistent evidence that editorial peer review may well increase the *readability* of papers in selected fields [2].

The quadrennial International Congress on the Scientific Evidence for the Contribution of Peer Review to Scientific Publication traces the evolution of evidence for the role of peer review. And yet, after seven Congresses over three decades, the evidence for peer review's contribution to editorial and publication processes appears to be thin at best. As of 2014, a compilation of 614 Congress abstracts [3] shows that 75% of these reports described observational studies; 18% intervention studies; and 7% opinion pieces.

The conclusion that emerges from these studies is that there is wide *belief* that peer review works to achieve improvement of a manuscript. However, in spite of numerous studies, the peer review process has not yielded to scientific analysis with the same precision of other aspects of biomedical science. Overbeke and Wager have proposed that the variability in findings of studies of peer review is probably because the research methods that have been employed do not serve complex social processes well [4]—a conclusion that will be recognizable to scholars of healthcare improvement science. While not necessarily a critically scientific conclusion, there is ultimately considerable support for the simple assertion that *it works because of faith in its effects* [5].

Although the published evidence for the efficacy of the aggregate of the complex social processes that we call peer review eludes precise scientific definition, its effectiveness might be said with confidence to be based substantially on its successful function as an improvement process. In sum, the paper that appears in a journal is the product of countless contributions—criticism, expert advice, suggestions, and counsel from colleagues along the way to publication. In that sense, it follows a path of classical principles of improvement—systematic assessments that ultimately contribute in formal and informal ways to its consistent improvement.

NINE RULES THAT CAN SERVE AS A GUIDE TO PEER REVIEW

Return with me to examine peer review specifically from the perspective of the *reviewer*. Wager and colleagues advanced three useful reviewer's questions. "Do I understand it? Do I believe it? Do I care?" [6]. Their utility lies in the fact that they speak directly to the expectations that you might reasonably assume are those of your ultimate reader.

Our resident trainees and faculty in the Dartmouth–Hitchcock LPMR writing collaborative invested several sessions in the development of a reviewer's systematic approach to a paper. While their goal was to develop a checklist for a formal journal review, these same elements can apply at the various sequential stages of a manuscript's development. The review by a peer-colleague at an early draft stage of a manuscript will be a simpler, more abbreviated process than that of a formal journal review, but the general principles can still apply.

Your manuscript's relentless progression is fueled by shared aims among colleagues. In this sense, it is an example of a classical improvement process—interplay between your aims as an author and the perspectives of interested and critical colleagues—co-authors, colleagues, or formal reviewers. I have framed here nine rules from a reviewer's perspective for use at any stage of a paper's development.

1. Identify and communicate your competence to review a particular paper. For example, this might be a patient's perspective, that of a system manager, a colleague with subject expertise or a clinician's perspective of a proposed improvement's contribution to clinical practice.
2. You of course should be mindful of any potential conflict of interest. Such a conflict might be substantial and disqualifying. More frequently, however, it is useful to simply consider your perspective and the ways that it might bias—even in small ways—your approach to the manuscript.
3. Base your perspective on a systematic reading of the *entire* paper. Try to read every section with an understanding of what appears to be the author's overall aim for the entire paper as well as the role for particular elements in achieving that aim.
4. Offer advice on the best fit for this paper in the literature. This can often offer considerations that the author might have overlooked.
5. Constantly develop a perspective of the paper's relative strengths and weaknesses. This requires serious reflection on the author's perceived intentions and messages. This is yet another opportunity for you to make contributions to the paper that go beyond wordsmithing and syntax, to focus on the author's success in achieving the paper's declared aims.

6. As a general rule, your review will be most useful if you can be specific—prioritizing opportunities for improvement. Accompany such comments by appropriate, specific suggestions.
7. It can be valuable to make use of a brief content checklist, for example, the SQUIRE 2.0 or PRISMA Publication Guidelines. Reviewing an improvement report with such a checklist at hand can serve to provide additional validity for your comments.
   Such a checklist will generally include at a minimum, an explicit improvement aim and study question; description of the intervention in sufficient detail that others might reproduce it in their settings; description of the study design that is intended to measure the impact of the intervention on outcomes; a description of results that appears valid as well as meaningful to a broad readership; and a conclusion regarding the implications of this work for patients and/or systems of care.
8. Examine carefully the tables and figures. Are they clear and is their relevance to the narrative in the text apparent? Can the legends stand alone as accurate and valuable explanations for the table or figure? Most importantly, do the tables and figures add value to the paper?
9. Finally, is the paper complete? Specifically, what might be missing?

RELATE PEER REVIEW EXPLICITLY TO YOUR AIMS AS AN AUTHOR

Returning again to your perspective as an author, peer review will take on greater importance as you approach journal submission. It will be useful at this point to consult your proposed journal's website for advice that it offers formal *reviewers*. Such reviewers' guidance offers valuable insights into a journal's editorial policies, and—in addition to your careful inspection of a journal's advice to *authors*—it can provide useful insights to help you refine a reasonable fit for your paper in this journal.

One final perspective of the relationship between author and reviewer: in our Dartmouth writing community, we emphasized a basic rule. The most generous contribution that you can offer a colleague is to make your review as critical as possible. A critical review at its best has the aim of making a manuscript as readable and valuable as possible before it receives the critical gaze of strangers, particularly journal reviewers. We concluded it is prudent to give less weight to the "friendly" reviewer who says a manuscript is flawless.

BECOME A PARTICIPANT IN THE EDITORIAL COMMUNITY AS A JOURNAL REVIEWER

There is yet another reviewer-related strategy that will contribute to your competence as an author. I encourage all authors to become a journal reviewer. It serves to introduce you to unique insights into the editorial community that are probably unavailable from any other perspective. It offers the opportunity to see what others are writing and submitting. It builds confidence to see how others' submissions look in their early stages.

Contact an editor of one of the journals that you read frequently and offer to be a reviewer. Specifically indicate the area of expertise that you bring to the journal. One of the constant challenges for editors is the development of a cadre of knowledgeable and willing reviewers, so you will be providing a substantial service to both the editor and the journal. It will contribute to a widening circle of writing colleagues—including the journal's editor.

Realize when you make this offer that a review is a time-consuming process, and the review must be provided in a timely way if it is to be useful to the editor. Your formal review of a manuscript for publication will usually take on average 2 to 5 hours. Usually when a review is requested, the journal staff communicates a defined deadline, often 2 to 3 weeks. Generally, the request for your review will include an abstract of the author's submitted paper. Needless to say, do not hesitate to turn down a request for a review that exceeds your expertise or field.

Contributing as an active reviewer in this scholarly community will provide you a fresh insider's perspective. A review is a generous gift to peers—for the submitting authors as well as your editor. Be a reviewer.

IN CONCLUSION...

Peer review describes the many interactions between you as an author and the many colleagues who will read your paper as it makes its way from first draft to its ultimate reader in a scholarly journal. Development of your competence as an effective reviewer will contribute substantially to your effectiveness as an author. Although the process has not yielded to scientific analysis, few doubt its contribution to the improvement and validity of the published scientific literature. I hope it is apparent that reviewing and writing inevitably converge in your development as a successful author.

REFERENCES

1. Kolb D. (1984). *Experiential Learning: Experience as the Source of Learning and Development.* Upper Saddle River, NJ: Prentice-Hall.
2. Jefferson T, Wager E, Davidoff F. Measuring the quality of editorial peer review. *JAMA* 2002;287:2786–2790.
3. Maliki M, von Elm E, Marusic A. Study design, publication outcome, and funding of research presented at International Congresses on Peer Review and Biomedical Publication. *JAMA* 2014;311:1065–1067.
4. Overbeke J, Wager E. (2003). The state of evidence: What we know and what we don't know about journal peer review. In Godlee F, Jefferson T, eds. *Peer Review in Health Sciences*, 2nd ed., pp. 45–61. London: BMJ Books.
5. Smith R. Peer review: A flawed process at the heart of science and journals. *J R Soc Med* 2006;99:178–182.
6. Wager E, Godlee F, Jefferson T. (2002). *How to Survive Peer Review.* London: BMJ Books.

CHAPTER 6
Develop a setting that facilitates your successful writing

CULTIVATE A SETTING THAT SUPPORTS YOUR WRITING

A community of healthcare improvement professionals continually supports their colleagues' effective writing for publication. To this end, try to cultivate your own formal opportunities for reviewing and revising that are part of the setting in which you and your colleagues assist each other to improve your writing.

"WHEN AND WHERE DO YOU WRITE?"

Such a setting requires constant attention to strategies that meet the challenge of fitting scholarly writing into a busy professional and personal life. Most productive authors I know have discovered that there is considerable efficiency to be found in a regular writing pattern. A set time and place will contribute to maintaining momentum in your writing. This usually works best if you can set aside a defined time that is reserved exclusively for writing. It will prove a constant challenge, but establishing that precious and jealously guarded writing time in your workday will go a long way toward making your writing process as effective as possible. Coupled with finding the time to write, establish a place that is reserved exclusively for your writing where you can write undistracted—set apart physically from other daily work.

Writing regularly will contribute to coping with the practical challenge of knowing where in a draft manuscript to resume writing when you next sit down to write. In this way, your personal writing sessions become a part of a continuum from one writing session to the next. One approach is to purposely end your writing each day in the middle of a task. Leave a thread or topic incomplete so as to hit the ground running right there at your next writing session. Having a thought ready to resume often means leaving the page while your concentration is working for you. However, those who do this routinely have discovered that it is easy to pick up that thread—that its momentum can be maintained from one writing session to the next.

When I was editor-in-chief of the journal *Quality and Safety in Health Care*, published in London, I would generally start writing at 5 A.M. in Cambridge, MA so I could synchronize with the London editorial staff that started work 5 hours ahead of my morning coffee. For efficiency and to take advantage of the expert professional support provided by the *BMJ* staff, I would set the clock for 2 hours of writing in the early moments of U.S. Eastern Standard Time.

I guess that means I am a lark. The world of authors is divided largely into larks—those who write most effectively upon arising in the morning—and owls—those who write most effectively after the sun has set. Maybe not the entire world, but in my instance, a practical effort at journal management soon turned into an opportunity to get a jump on the day by writing when I, a confirmed lark, was most effective.

It is said that Richard Selzer, the Yale surgeon-author, learned early in his writing career the value of using early pre-dawn hours for writing. He would set his clock for the middle of the night to write for several hours in the quiet of his study. His approach to juxtaposing time for writing against a busy surgeon's life eschewed all other activities at that moment to maintain this remarkable focus on writing.

A SUNDAY MORNING EMAIL

In an effort to address this question for discussion with my Dartmouth writing collaborative, one Sunday morning in 2010 I sent an email message to a handful of writer/clinician/educator colleagues. I simply asked them, "When and where do you write?" I deliberately selected successful authors who appeared to me to be highly productive writers but I also knew they were busy healthcare professionals with demanding day jobs.

As it turned out this query clearly tapped into a vein. I was surprised when I received responses from all of them—almost all before sundown the same day! Four have given me permission to share their responses, which I do here *verbatim.*

Harlan Krumholtz is a cardiologist, researcher, and educator at Yale Medical School in New Haven, CT. He is the author of over 800 peer-reviewed scholarly reports and newspaper commentaries.

He responded,

When I was earlier in my career, I would start writing late in the evening when we finally were able to get the kids to sleep. We have four—and our style is fairly permissive—so sometimes that might have been close to 11—sometimes earlier. The house was active and it was too much fun to force them to go to sleep earlier. Then I would stay up late often—I never found time to write during the day because the days were always packed. Now the kids are mostly grown (one at home now—a soph in hs) and that has changed but professionally I have much more to occupy me and pull me from writing. I find that I spend so much time keeping up with email traffic—much of it related to projects or mentoring or tasks such as journal reviews/journal editing/promotion letters/grant reviews and so on—that I am challenged to sequester quiet time to write—so I just do my best to get ahead of the urgent so I can focus on the less urgent but, to me, equally important task of writing papers and editorials and, now, blogs and op-eds. I usually get enough ahead to do that at night or sometime on the weekend. I feel that writing is so important—it forces a need to be precise in language and logic—and remains a highly effective means to disseminate new knowledge and ideas. But it remains a challenge and what is urgent and important has grown—and email is a blessing and a curse.

Atul Gawande is a researcher, teacher, and surgeon at Harvard-affiliated Brigham and Women's Hospital in Boston, MA. He has published extensively in the *New Yorker*, as well as academic peer-reviewed reports and best-selling books such as *Complications: A Surgeon's Notes on an Imperfect Science* and *Being Mortal: Illness, Medicine and What Matters in the End*.

He wrote simply, I wish it were regular. I write more randomly, between cases, weekends, whatever, wherever I can find a hospital computer or laptop or legal pad and whenever I can free up time from other commitments."

Bob Wachter is the Chair of Medicine at the University of California, San Francisco School of Medicine. He is author of numerous best-selling books including The Digital Doctor: Hope, Hype and Harm at the Dawn of Medicine's Computer Age and over 250 scholarly articles. For years he has been a consistent and industrious blogger on the frequently visited site, Wachter's World, which is now a part of the Hospital Leader, the official blog of the Society of Hospital Medicine.

He responded,

> Boy, I wish I was disciplined enough to write every day. I don't, and don't really think I can, between all the other things on my plate. My only daily ritual is reading the Times—I don't go to sleep before I've done that.
>
> I have committed myself to about one blog post per week, and have been pretty good about keeping up that pace for 3 years. So I block about half a day sometime each week to get this done, though there are times when this plan flies out the window—a new issue hits and I want to get a blog out more quickly, and I just find the time.
>
> For my blogs, I find that the average one takes about 3–5 hours to write (including the research, finding the links), and another hour to post (loading in the links, etc). Each piece averages about 1200 words, though some are longer (for example, my most recent one, on airplane emergencies, is 2600). One rule is never to post on the day I write it. So I try to get it written early in the day, look at it after a few hours break, sometimes have my significant other (who's an accomplished author) read it over, and then save it in the posting too—but then to sleep on it and post it the next morning. I find that overnight break

is crucial—I virtually always find things I want to change, ranging from typos to more major changes.

When I'm writing a book, I'm pretty religious about taking every Friday off and going to my favorite little cafe for the entire day. Although I tend to check my email every hour or so, on those days, I really try to discipline myself to only check about twice in the day, and to limit my web browsing to things I really need. If I'm really serious, I won't log onto the web at all.

Writing more traditional articles, who knows? I just find the time when I can, often nights and weekends. But here too, having a full day to write is the key for me. Some writers do well in 1 hour blocks/day; I really prefer longer blocks of time. Somehow, I do have the stamina to write for 8–10 hours, especially if I'm jazzed by the topic.

As every writer knows, the key is to push yourself to get something down on "paper"—once it's there, the editing part tends to be relatively easy.

Ken Ludmerer is a medical historian, educator, and practicing specialist in internal medicine at Washington University School of Medicine in St. Louis, MO. He is author of several insightful books, including *Let Me Heal: The Opportunity to Preserve Excellence in American Medicine.*

He wrote,

I do my serious writing at my home office. It's quiet, I'm able to achieve a deeper level of concentration because there are fewer distractions, I have an unusually fine library on American medical education for reference, and I'm able to get to the medical center quickly if necessary. I find that I need lengthy blocks of time to write effectively—a few hours minimum. I precede the actual writing (pen to paper, finger to keyboard) with considerable thinking. Before writing a book, I want to have an outline of the entire project before writing anything. Before writing a chapter or article, I figure out in my mind what I want to say before I sit down and try to say it.

When I write depends on whether I'm on or off service. I'm on the conventional "investigator" or "academic" track, which allows me considerable time for research and writing. I like to say that when my physician-scientist colleagues are in the lab, I'm in the library. Typically, I attend on in-patient internal medicine four months a year. If I'm on service, I might get a few hours done a day. If I'm off service, I have ample time, sometimes an entire day if there are no meetings, conferences, student or resident counseling, administrative duties, professional obligations (reviewing manuscripts and so forth), etc.

I was staggered by the generous wisdom that these colleagues were willing to share! The dominant message that literally flew off the screen was their passion for writing. Each clearly had discovered the enormous reward that writing offers in their professional and personal lives. A reassuring (and humbling!) theme is that no one is afforded more than the same 24-hour day that you and I share. How they crafted their professional and personal lives to commit to effective writing resonated profoundly with my busy trainee and faculty colleagues as I suspect it does with you.

HOW WOULD YOU ANSWER MY SUNDAY MORNING EMAIL?

When I explored this same question with the Dartmouth trainees and faculty, a wide variety of responses emerged. Regardless of the details, the predominant response was that all participants stopped and reflected deeply on where writing fits in their lives. Importantly, most did indeed follow this discussion with adjustments to their own writing habits.

There was such grace and wisdom in the messages from these busy colleagues that Sunday in 2010. I urge you to find your own lessons here. Take the time to reflect on when and where you write. Perhaps more importantly, how does your reflection lead to more effective and productive writing? What modifications do you need to craft for a more systematic approach to your own writing?

WHY ESTABLISH A STRATEGY FOR REGULAR WRITING AND REVIEWING WITH COLLEAGUES?

In addition to identifying the time and place for your own personal writing, consider a similar strategy for regular writing and reviewing together with colleagues. Such a strategy can take the form of a formal writing workshop, a self-organizing writing collaborative, or a focused writing tutorial. Whatever you call it, its overriding aim should be to provide a context where colleagues support each other's work by providing supportive and constructive feedback for each other's draft manuscripts. Again the important issue here is to develop a regular setting for supportive, timely, and effective collegial peer review.

This comes back to the fundamental premise for your writing for publication. You write to be read. Development of a formal setting for sharing manuscripts with critical, collaborative reviewers and readers will serve as a valuable step in establishing a continuum for work on your own draft manuscript on its way to your ultimate journal reader.

EXAMPLES OF FORMAL WRITING GROUPS

Our experiences with numerous formal writing groups—from students and resident trainees to seasoned healthcare professionals—provide examples of the wide variety of settings that can facilitate writing with colleagues. Consider these four different examples to see if there are elements that might contribute to your organizing a setting for systematic writing with colleagues.

The first example is the Dartmouth Hitchcock Leadership and Preventive Medicine Residency (LPMR) writing program. It was developed and revised over a 5-year period (2008–2012) and consisted of 2-year cohorts of doctors-in-training and their faculty. The aim of the program was to develop competency in writing for the scholarly healthcare improvement literature. The trainees came from a variety of medical specialties. All trainees combined preventive medicine with their clinical specialty—18 different combinations including internal medicine and its sub-specialties, family medicine, surgery, psychiatry, ob-gyn pediatrics, and others.

The residency was established to develop physicians to be skilled in healthcare system improvement as well as leaders of change for improvement. To address the topic of writing for publication, the trainees and their faculty met formally every month for 90-minute writing sessions. An explicit curriculum was developed that explored the challenges of writing, the daunting task of sharing one's writing with others, and the various strategies for helping colleagues with their own writing. The sessions emphasized the roles of colleagues as co-authors and reviewers rather than placing an explicit emphasis on expert coaching. (Please see the Appendix for an extensive summary of the curriculum.)

All residents conducted at least one extensive, in-depth systems improvement initiative, and each resident successfully prepared one or more publications based on this improvement research. The number of peer-reviewed reports of improvement initiatives that were successfully published within 2 years of completing the program serves as an example of the possibilities for such a program. Assessment of the initial 4 resident cohorts during the first 5 years of the writing program showed that 11 of 24 resident trainees achieved peer-reviewed publication of at least one or more reports of their improvement work.

A *faculty* writing collaborative offers a second example of a strategy for writing effectively with peers. After the first year of the LPMR writing program, the faculty became aware of their own unique writing challenges and learning needs. This led to the development of a separate self-organizing monthly session, which was developed exclusively for faculty. Their writing skills were generally better developed than those of the trainees, but they had more compelling career-related motivation to publish.

The faculty group agreed to three principal aims: greater publication productivity, enhanced effectiveness as teachers of scholarly writing, and taking full advantage of the opportunity for reflection that scholarly writing offers for one's professional and personal life. In addition, they agreed to three simple rules to maintain this focus. Each participant committed to work actively on a draft manuscript, to write at least 3 hours a week, and to participate in the monthly 90-minute faculty writing session.

A third example of convening like-minded authors is provided by a web-based writing workshop for academic leaders that was supported by the Institute for Healthcare Improvement. The participants were predominantly senior academic leaders from diverse academic institutions with considerable experience in publication in other biomedical disciplines, but they were all relatively new to healthcare improvement science. The web sessions among these workshop participants shed light on their own unique challenges for colleagues writing together. For example, the variation in authority gradients among participants across these institutions brought unanticipated challenges when these leaders convened in the leveling environment of the writing webinars. This culture contrasted with the homogeneity among the LPMR resident trainees. A similarity to the trainee's writing initiative, however, became apparent early in the program. Greater academic experience in no way assures participants' comfort in sharing early manuscript drafts with colleagues.

The final example is a national writing initiative that was convened for selected co-author teams. All participants came to this initiative specifically committed to achieving publication of their improvement work related to their care of persons with the chronic disease, Cystic Fibrosis (CF). The teams were selected from the extensive national CF community of researchers, improvers, and educators [1].

Supported by the Cystic Fibrosis Foundation, the aims of the initiative were to provide an opportunity for a variety of colleagues to publish in the scholarly healthcare improvement literature, raise the visibility of good CF research, and identify important contributions that this work might provide to the care of persons with other chronic illnesses and in different types of academic settings [2].

A formal abstract selection process winnowed 47 submissions to 9 teams that were selected to participate. These teams worked aggressively toward their agreed aims. Five months were devoted to their writing. This consisted of three webinars and one 2-day face-to-face workshop. Five more months were devoted to the submission and review processes, which led finally to the *BMJ Quality and Safety* supplement, *Ten Years of Improvement Innovation in Cystic Fibrosis Care* [3]. In addition to the manuscripts that were developed by the selected teams, invited editorials and commentaries were included in the final 15 papers that were the product of this initiative [3].

SIX STEPS TO ESTABLISHING YOUR OWN LOCAL WRITING COLLABORATIVE

What might you learn from a review of these experiences as you contemplate developing your own writing group? While these examples were widely different in format, resources, professional participants, and aims, they shared overarching themes.

Common to all was the expectation that participants would regularly share writing products at any stage of a manuscript's development. All groups developed their own clear aims, and they were most effective if the participants themselves determined those aims. The writing and reviewing processes were served by Plan-Do-Study-Act improvement cycles to test small improvements to assure that participants in the writing group remained on track with productive writing from meeting to meeting.

On the other hand, there was a unique culture that developed in each writing group. For example, medical trainees came at writing together differently from nursing trainees or senior medical faculty. Homogeneity is not a requirement, but mindfulness of differences among professional cultures will serve well as you work to establish a formal writing community.

Based on these experiences, here are six suggested steps to establishing your own local writing group.

1. Recruit colleagues who agree—indeed, commit—to write regularly and share writing products.
2. By consensus, establish a defined meeting interval, time, and place. It can be accomplished with as few as a pair of colleagues who meet weekly in a local coffee shop [Okumura, MJ. personal communication] or a larger community of like-minded authors who convene monthly. The point is to commit to the set time and place.
3. Employ relentless peer review. Work in pairs or trios to trade roles as author and reviewer. Agree to a few simple rules that include generous but blunt criticism.
4. Consider the added dividend of developing session topics and readings that can foster continuous learning about the science of improvement, the evolving scholarly literature, and editorial expectations.
5. Rotate the task of session leader among participants. The leader picks the session's topic. The agenda can be as simple as each participant presenting his or her current greatest writing challenge, to everyone writing spontaneously on the same topic. Keep expectations and pre-work assignments clear and simple.
6. Assert a measure of self-discipline for writing sessions. Start immediately with writing at each session. There will be an appeal in finding topics and activities other than writing when you gather. Avoid the temptation to use sessions as social events.

MAINTAINING MOMENTUM IN YOUR LOCAL WRITING GROUP

It is easy to initiate a writing collaborative—such as the examples above—but it is harder to keep it going. Keep track of successful publications. Be sure to celebrate success.

On the other hand, be alert to signs of flagging momentum—for example, dropping attendance, uninspired session leadership, or reduced individual commitment to finding new writing projects. These challenges can be met by addressing each as it occurs. If necessary, consider devoting a session to identifying sources of such speed bumps.

To maintain interest, consider inviting external "consultants" to occasional writing sessions. Examples include the local IRB chair, a critical colleague who is unfamiliar with writing for healthcare improvement, or colleagues who can bring new epistemologies and different methodologies to the group. While institutional improvement experts can contribute substantial supporting roles, there can be great value in seasoning the mix with colleagues from related fields such as management, sociology, health services research, bioethics, etc. All can bring fresh perspectives to the challenges of effective scholarly writing.

Remember to keep your institutional senior leadership aware of the outcomes of your writing initiative. A group of colleagues who gather regularly to support each other's professional writing contributes to the work of department or division leadership in their obligation to stimulate scholarly publication. Moreover, keep leaders mindful of the additional dividend that is provided by colleagues who mentor each other.

When the opportunity presents itself, find ways to develop creative financial support for the writing initiative. Ask. As an example, a Visiting Professor initiative was implemented during the second year of the Dartmouth faculty writing group with support from the unit chief. He recognized the contribution that such a Visiting Professor initiative brought to the larger academic community as well as the positive reflection among colleagues that it shed on his unit. The institution hosted four nationally acknowledged improvement scholars and editors. Each visitor provided a series of conferences with residents, meetings with the faculty, Grand Rounds, and an institution-wide writing Master Class. Their participation provided both external validation for scholarly improvement publication as well as fresh and diverse perspectives from national leaders in the healthcare improvement field. As an unanticipated dividend, durable, productive mentorships developed among visitors and selected Dartmouth residents and faculty.

WHY WE WRITE

Writing and publishing is an integral part of the work of healthcare improvement. Nevertheless, maintaining a professional environment that supports your writing is not simple. Such an environment is yet another element in your professional life that is designed to make your improvement work more accessible through its publication for the wider benefit of patients. In its most basic form, reviewing and revising is a process where colleagues are constantly assisting each other to find transparency and clarity. Perhaps even more importantly, the reflective nature of writing—alone and with colleagues—offers insights into your work and, perhaps at a deeper level, clarity about your identity as a health professional.

REFERENCES

1. Stevens DP, Marshall BC. Healthcare improvement is incomplete until it is published: The cystic fibrosis initiative to support scholarly publication. *BMJ Qual Saf* 2014;23:i104–i107.
2. Stevens DP, Marshall BC. A decade of healthcare improvement in cystic fibrosis: Lessons for other chronic diseases. *BMJ Qual Saf* 2014;23:i1–i2.
3. Stevens DP, Marshall BC, Supplement Eds. Ten years of improvement innovation in cystic fibrosis care. *BMJ Qual Saf* 2014; (Suppl 1) 23:i1–i107.

CHAPTER 7

The essential role for context in your healthcare improvement report

WHY IS CONTEXT SO IMPORTANT?

Healthcare improvement is a social process. It requires that people cooperate and agree to work toward shared goals. It challenges them to change behavior. The improvement interventions themselves, for example, checklists, bundles, or formulas, are essential elements of an improvement initiative, but they are at best only half the process. Understanding and communicating the complexities of context, and how it interacts with these elements—the unique social backdrop as well as the physical setting in which your initiative is implemented— is essential for your reader's full understanding of your improvement initiative.

Getting this right requires your analysis of how your initiative's context can recognizably relate to that of your reader. Specifically, how might your analysis help your reader identify local issues that can contribute to his or her own success? The *improvement strategies* are usually the constant and replicable elements of similar initiatives from setting to setting. In many ways, the strategies are the easy part. On the other hand, communicating your initiative's unique *context* is a challenge that plays an essential role in conveying your new improvement knowledge to your reader [1]. This chapter will explore how you can effectively identify, analyze, and report these critical contextual elements.

DEVELOP AN EFFECTIVE APPROACH TO COMMUNICATING CONTEXT

This matter of discerning and describing effectively the uniquely relevant contextual elements in *your* particular initiative will add substantially to your paper's contribution to advancing healthcare improvement. Nevertheless, it is one of the most daunting aspects of writing to improve healthcare.

We will explore different sources for an extensive catalog of contextual elements and how they have been analyzed in patient safety and healthcare improvement literature. We will also examine practical strategies for your communicating the relevant new knowledge and insights that can be found in systematic observation and reflection on your improvement initiative.

DESCRIBE THE SETTING, BUT DIG DEEPER

In most clinical research, context is held constant so that the effect of a proposed treatment or medication can be validly attributed to the procedure or agent being tested [2]. The science of healthcare improvement—and therefore you as a healthcare improvement author—has an added burden of establishing the evidence for identifying for the reader those parts of the context that actually contributed to the observed success for an improvement initiative. In addition to the "where," the important parts of context are the "how" and "why." Therein lies the importance of the author's careful reflection and study to provide a measure of the empirical evidence for the relevant contextual elements, separating them out from all the potentially lurking confounders in a healthcare setting.

It calls for more than a description of the physical setting—for example, the academic or financial characteristics of a hospital system or its geographic setting. While these practical details are generally relevant, they are not the elements that lead the reader to grasp the full implications of a successful (or unsuccessful) initiative.

"WHAT THEN ARE THE ESSENTIAL ELEMENTS OF CONTEXT THAT YOU ALWAYS NEED TO REPORT?"

When we wrestled with understanding context in our Dartmouth writing collaborative, the residents invariably moved to a question, something like, "Well, what then are the elements of context that we always need to report?" Together we concluded the answer is neither simple nor totally reassuring.

There is no mandatory checklist of essential elements of "context" that must go into every healthcare improvement paper. However, it is useful to examine systematic reviews of recent improvement publications that probed this question—focused specifically on accumulating contextual elements that appear to play meaningful roles. These reviews provide useful perspectives, which may be relevant to your own careful analysis of context and its apparent contribution to your improvement initiative.

SUMMARY STUDIES THAT EMPHASIZE CULTURE, LEADERSHIP, AND SYSTEM CONNECTIVITY

Three studies offer different approaches to providing pragmatic analyses of the role of relevant contextual elements in effective improvement initiatives. The first employs an expert consensus process. The second is a critical review of the available empirical evidence for context in the improvement literature. The third is a systematic review that dissected in detail particular elements that facilitated the spread of innovation.

The consensus approach was used by a team of investigators at RAND in collaboration with an international group of improvement and patient safety experts. They convened a so-called technical expert panel—on which I served with 21 others—supported by funding from the U.S. Agency for Healthcare Research and Quality (AHRQ). The goal of the study was to develop a taxonomy of the elements of context that appeared to contribute to the successful implementation of five selected patient safety practices [3]. The specific safety practices that were analyzed included: a universal protocol to avoid wrong-site surgery; medication reconciliation—the practice of assuring that the patient is taking the same medications across various care settings; computer assisted decision systems for clinicians; reduction of patient falls; and checklists to reduce blood stream infections.

The initial consensus concluded that context is generally inadequately described in most scholarly patient safety reports. Failure to implement an accepted safety practice may not be because of ignorance of the evidence-based technique, but rather the inability to discern and employ the complex clinical and social changes that appear to be required for implementing the safety initiative.

That being said, the panel accumulated a total of 42 contextual elements. They were divided—some might argue, wedged—into four broad domains. The first domain lumped together safety culture, teamwork, and leadership. The second domain included structural organizational characteristics, for example, size, organizational complexity, and financial status. Third, external factors were grouped to include financial or performance incentives as well as patient safety performance regulations. Finally, the panel invoked the availability of management and implementation tools, which formed a grab bag of elements such as internal incentives and internal organizational incentives.

A second perspective for discerning relevant contextual elements was provided by a systematic literature review conducted by Kaplan and colleagues at Cincinnati Children's Medical Center. Their aim was to identify reports that described empirical *evidence* for the influence of contextual elements on improvement initiatives [4]. Of over 15,000 potentially useful reports, 41 papers were identified as providing sufficiently critical evidence in a way that was useful for this purpose. A critical analysis of this relatively small group of papers yielded 66 contextual elements, which these authors grouped in five categories.

In their first category were organizational issues. These include top management leadership, the maturity of an organization's involvement with quality improvement, and the presence of a culture supportive of improvement. The second category included institutional quality improvement development and support. The emphasis here is on important practical elements such as data management systems, funding, as well as sufficient professional time for improvement initiatives. Of note, workforce development for improvement was included in this category but was found to be insufficiently effective as an isolated element. Alone it was not highly correlated with success. The third category described microsystem characteristics. Microsystem level leadership and a microsystem's capability to change were highly correlated with success. Fourth, a substantial contribution was identified for selected characteristics of quality improvement teams. Of particular importance was team leadership and quality improvement capability. The final category was the identification of the relevance of the improvement initiative to the organization's overall goals.

A third source for contextual elements was the early seminal work of Greenhalgh and colleagues [5], together with the subsequent work of Damschroder et al. [6]. We examined Greenhalgh's extensive systematic review that focused on spread of innovation in Chapter 1. It described an important role for leadership with specific emphasis on so-called champions, as well as a profound impact for selected cultural elements. They demonstrated insightfully how these elements served to facilitate successful spread in some settings but their absence in other settings resulted in those settings' inability to host the same improvement and innovation.

A Consolidated Framework for Implementation Research (CFIR) was developed on the foundation laid by Greenhalgh's conceptual models [6]. This pragmatic summary boiled down an extensive body of theory to practical elements that included, for example, leadership that has the long view, organizational culture, cost incentives, peer pressure, tension for change, and effective planning.

REPORTING CONTEXT: CULTURE

Prominent among the findings from all of these summary studies were rich and innovative approaches to the complex issue of organizational *Culture* as context. All reviews described similar elements that contributed to success. Prominent examples among these were safety culture, innovativeness, teamwork, readiness to change, recognized need for change [3], creativity, risk-taking, stability, and a supportive learning culture [4].

REPORTING CONTEXT: LEADERSHIP

A second broad category that emerges from these studies is *Leadership*. Leadership is typically considered to be under the aegis of senior organization leaders such as CEOs, Nursing Directors, Chief Medical Officers, or Clinical Department Chairs or Chiefs. Of importance, however, was the finding that there are leaders at the individual unit level in a health system that contribute substantially to facilitating or impeding implementation of healthcare improvement initiatives. For example, nurse-managers of patient care units such as an ambulatory care clinic or an intensive care unit hold substantial day-to-day authority over patient management. Their buy-in to any substantial change in processes or care strategies is essential. In this regard, leadership strategies at the improvement and the patient care team levels were central to many effective improvement initiatives.

Kaplan et al. described three consistent findings that address how leadership is a relevant contextual element. These observations were not necessarily intuitive. Or are they? On the one hand, they found a positive contribution for top leaders that communicate vision, strategy, and expectations. On the other hand, top-down planning by leadership alone was not an effective element. A third element— probably the strongest contextual impact for leadership—was top management's *active participation* in improvement activities. So, leaders who communicate their vision and expectations are helpful, while top-down planning is not so helpful; and leaders' active participation in improvement is very helpful. On reflection, this probably holds no surprises for most readers.

REPORTING CONTEXT: ORGANIZATIONAL CONNECTIVITY

There was also much contained in these studies about the broad contextual category of *Organizational Connectivity*. Examples included the effective role for microsystems in the larger concentric rings of other microsystems and macrosystems—and their complex interactions. Effective teams integrate culture, leadership, and connectivity on the ground level.

Reports of healthcare improvement initiatives generally do not describe the dozens of negotiations and meetings required for an improvement initiative. Consider the relevant care units or the policy committees such as those that oversee hospital records or institutional pharmacy rules. Stephen Liu, now a hospitalist leader at Dartmouth–Hitchcock Medical Center, describes having to meet with upwards of 20 committees and institutional leaders to negotiate a measure of consensus for a study designed to implement a standard of care for initiation of antibiotic therapy for community-acquired pneumonia [7]. Often the authority and influence of such groups or individuals require repeated meetings or informal discussions including hallway consultations or cafeteria encounters [Liu, S, personal communication]. Such details generally do not find their way into healthcare improvement reports. Should they be included?

TO COMPLICATE MATTERS, CONTEXT DOES NOT REMAIN STATIC

One more consideration just to complicate your author's task further: as an improvement initiative unfolds, changes inevitably evolve in the context consequent to the initiative's impact on the institutional setting. You must try to accommodate these so-called reflexive changes in the description of your local context. Reflexiveness must be carefully analyzed and reported as yet another contextual detail that underlies the dissemination of a successful process to improve care.

COMMUNICATING A PERSPECTIVE OF CONTEXT IN YOUR MANUSCRIPT

All of which brings us back to how you might take advantage of the questions that our writing collaborative trainees raised about a useful "list" of relevant contextual elements. The abbreviated overview of contextual elements above (see Table 7.1) boils down to organizational culture, leadership, the role of peer interaction, and the ability of members of a healthcare organization to work collaboratively, specifically, in inter-professional teams. And yet, as Kaplan and colleagues found in the articles identified by their review, listing these categories is just the beginning. These elements frequently converge with regard to their

Table 7.1 Examples of contextual elements that can contribute to healthcare improvement initiatives

Culture

- Maturity of an organization's involvement with quality improvement
- Presence of a culture supportive of improvement
- Quality improvement capability
- Safety culture
- Teamwork
- Innovativeness
- Readiness to change
- Recognized need for change
- Tension for change
- Stability
- Creativity
- Risk-taking
- Peer pressure
- Supportive learning culture
- Internal organizational incentives
- Microsystem capability to change
- Team level quality improvement capability

Leadership

- Management leadership style
- Top leaders who *communicate* vision, strategy, and expectations
- Involvement of top leadership in improvement initiatives
- Leadership that has the long view
- Clinical Unit level leadership
- Emphasis on team leadership
- Microsystem level leadership

Organizational Connectivity

- Microsystem connectivity for efficient, safe patient care
- Relevance of the improvement initiative to the overall organization's goals
- Data management systems
- Internal organizational incentives

(Continued)

Table 7.1 (*Continued*) Examples of contextual elements that can contribute to healthcare improvement initiatives

- Organizational complexity
- Response to external performance and financial incentives
- Broad awareness of patient safety performance guidelines

Source: Summarized from a consensus process reported by Taylor, SL et al., *BMJ Qual Saf,* 20, 611–617, 2011 and a systematic review by Kaplan, SL et al., *Milbank Q,* 88, 500–559, 2010. These are but summary examples. The reader is urged to explore the detailed lists of contextual elements that will be found in these references.

relative contributions to an initiative—for example, collaboration is very difficult without an organizational culture that fosters teams and mutual respect across professional disciplines.

Your identification of contextual elements such as culture, leadership, and organizational connectivity along with other relevant elements in your institution requires your careful and systematic observation. Now, how do you make sense of these observations? And finally, how do you capture this sense-making in your report? Kaveh Shojania, the current editor-in-chief of *BMJ Quality and Safety,* and I summarized a five-point approach to reporting context [8].

1. Diligently drill down on the elements that contributed to your success.
2. Take a stab at what you consider the empiric evidence for their contribution.
3. What is your theory for this? Set this against the backdrop of context in the literature. Remember this is your work. Who is better positioned to dig into this than you? It calls for your thoughtful *retrospective* analysis as you write your paper.
4. Elaborate explicitly on the elements that you consider absolutely essential to your success. This is the news in your report [1]. It is the core. What happened in your experience that supports this conclusion?
5. Remember to relate this to *your readers'* contexts—*writing mindful of your reader.* Such mindfulness will add immensely to the potential value, as well as readability and interest for your paper.

WHERE DOES YOUR DESCRIPTION OF CONTEXT BELONG IN YOUR PAPER?

Where does the description of context belong in the formal structure of your improvement paper? The short answer is everywhere that it readily fits. That includes a careful description of the local problem that was identified for improvement in your Introduction as well as a relevant description of context as it fits in Methods. When reporting the Results, reflect in depth on context's role in the outcomes. Moreover, give careful consideration in Limitations to how selected contextual elements in this intervention might (or might not) be found in the reader's setting. The recently revised SQUIRE 2.0 Publication Guidelines list a number of places you might consider [9]. Write fully mindful of the contextual challenges that you encountered and give particular attention to how they might be relevant to your reader's setting.

THE CONTEXT IS INDEED YOUR NEWS

Paul Bate has written eloquently, "The context is everything" [10]. When the Dartmouth trainees and faculty in the LPMR writing collaborative drilled down relentlessly on examples of successful reports, they found this same truth that lay beneath the headlines in a successful report. The real news for the reader was communicated in the unique complexities of its social and cultural context. More often than not in a healthcare improvement article, *the context is the news* [1].

Now it is imperative to go further still—the description for your reader of the *study* of your improvement initiative. Central to your report is the question of how these two fundamental ingredients—*your unique context* and the *improvement intervention*—interact to lead to better care. In the next chapter, we will explore that complex set of elements that flesh out the full meaning of this new knowledge that your initiative offers your reader.

REFERENCES

1. Stevens DP. The context is the "news" in healthcare improvement case reports. *Qual Saf Health Care* 2010;19:162–163.
2. Davidoff F. Heterogeneity is not always noise: Lessons from improvement. *JAMA* 2009;302(23):2580–2586.

3. Taylor SL, Dy S, Foy R, et al. What context features might be important determinants of the effectiveness of patient safety interventions? *BMJ Qual Saf* 2011;20:611–617.

4. Kaplan HC, Brady PW, Dritz MC, et al. The influence of context on improvement success in Health Care: A systematic review of the literature. *Milbank Q* 2010;88:500–559.

5. Greenhalgh T, Robert G, Macfarlane F, et al. Diffusion of innovations in service organizations: Systematic review and recommendations. *Milbank Q* 2004;82:581–629.

6. Damschroder LJ, Aron DC, Keith RE, et al. Fostering implementation of health services research findings into practice: A consolidated framework for advancing implementation science. *Implementation Sci* 2009;4:50.

7. Liu SK, Homa KA, Butterly JR, et al. Improving the simple, complicated, and complex realities of community-acquired pneumonia. *Qual Saf Health Care* 2009;18:93–98.

8. Stevens DP, Shojania KG. Tell me about the context, and more. *BMJ Qual Saf* 2011;20:557–559.

9. Ogrinc G, Davies L, Goodman D, et al. SQUIRE 2.0 (Standards for QUality Improvement Reporting Excellence): Revised publication guidelines from a detailed consensus process. *BMJ Qual Saf* 2016;25:986–992.

10. Bate P. *The Context is Everything*. Perspectives on Context. The Health Foundation 2014. http://www.health.org.uk/sites/health/files/PerspectivesOnContextBateContextIsEverything.pdf. Accessed September 29, 2017.

CHAPTER 8
Reporting the study of your improvement

THE STUDY OF YOUR IMPROVEMENT

Early reports of healthcare improvement focused principally on description of the improvement intervention. As healthcare improvement science has evolved, healthcare improvement professionals have come to recognize that there is another layer of analysis for a critical report of an improvement intervention—that layer includes your insightful *study of the process* [1,2]. What does this new layer of analysis contribute to advancing healthcare improvement?

Your over-riding obligation in writing to improve healthcare is to bring your reader to the point where he or she sees how the initiative might be successfully implemented in that reader's healthcare setting. Elements that will flesh this out include your insightful perspective of the rationale for your undertaking the initiative, the relevant program theory that might underlie this rationale, the strength of evidence that supports the conclusion that the changes that you observed were actually due to your improvement intervention, and the so-called *ex post* assessment of why your particular initiative was (or was not) successfully put into practice. We will explore these elements in your healthcare improvement manuscript, where they fit best, and how to know you have provided sufficient insight into these elements for your reader to make good use of your report for the benefit of further healthcare improvement. This is a tall order for you as author.

STUDY OF THE IMPROVEMENT: REPORTING THE RATIONALE THAT UNDERLIES YOUR IMPROVEMENT INITIATIVE

An insightful report of the theory that underlies an improvement initiative is fundamental to your reader's understanding of the place where you believe your initiative sits in the continuum of healthcare improvement [3]. Your rationale generally belongs upfront in the Introduction. Providing your reader an analysis of the rationale has also been called "reason-giving" [4].

Akin to the hypothesis development that is a familiar and mandatory component of biomedical research, the rationale for a healthcare improvement initiative has been framed effectively in terms of theory development [3]. Davidoff et al. [4] have made the case that insightful theory development serves to build the science of improvement by going beyond the author's intuition—contributing fundamentally to new learning for the benefit of patients and health systems.

THE CYSTIC FIBROSIS CARE NETWORK: A CASE STUDY FOR REPORTING RATIONALE

The story of the Cystic Fibrosis Care Center Network provides a case study for the contribution to new knowledge of clearly defined program theory. The chronicle of the CF Network's 50-year experience is a stunning story of relentless improvement in survival and life expectancy in persons with this serious chronic disease. Initially considered a life-threatening childhood illness, persons with CF now can expect to live well into adulthood. CF care has been marked by consistent adherence to theory that has anchored the development of the CF Center Network, which now consists of over 130 CF Care Centers.

The Network was launched in 1960. An underlying rationale for the Network improvement strategies was developed by broad consensus. It spoke to adherence to "sustained leadership for change, shared quality improvement approaches across all Centers, incorporation of people with CF and their families in the improvement work, identifying and enabling CF care best practices, and providing decision-support for care teams" [5]. As the Network initiative developed, individual program strategy dictated program level theory for specific strategies that addressed, for example, improvement in nutrition [6], controlling infection [7], and preserving adequate pulmonary function [8]. While consistent attention to both overarching network level theory as well as program level theory served the improvement initiatives, their lucid articulation was essential for the spread of improvement widely across the network of CF care centers.

Davidoff et al. have suggested a useful analytic strategy that might help you identify the theory that underlies your initiative [4]. They suggest an approach that literally follows a path dictated by "If…, then…, so that…." For example, hypothetical application of such a frame to the cystic fibrosis chronic care initiative might look like the following. Stay with me as we walk through this. *If* a vision that focused on exemplary CF care could be provided by Network leadership, *then* development of exemplary standards of care and dissemination of health outcome data—for example, by implementation of an effective registry—might be realized, *so that* key strategies and opportunities for improvement could be achieved, *so that* persons with CF might achieve better nutrition, improved pulmonary function, and better pancreatic function, *so that* children and adolescents attain normal growth and development, patients and families have strengthened, well-informed collaboration with clinicians, exacerbations of illness are detected early and patients are returned to normal function earlier.

Each of the many local CF initiatives was driven by adherence to overarching Network strategies—some more successfully than others. Study of the most successful initiatives provided benchmarking opportunities for other centers, powered by adherence to consistent maintenance of accessible and reliable registry data. It is fair to say that the complex evolution of theory-based CF care strategies also goes beyond CF care improvement *per se* to offer lessons for other chronic diseases [9].

Think carefully about the underlying theory for your improvement initiative. At the risk of being overly formulaic, another way to test your rationale is to hold it up to the criteria suggested by the authors of SQUIRE 2.0 AND StaRI Publication Guidelines. The authors of the StaRI Guidelines ask for your hypothesis with particular attention to background information and a rationale for how the implementation might work [10]. The authors of SQUIRE 2.0 offer a somewhat more granular mini-checklist to define your rationale—"informal or formal frameworks, models, concepts and/or theories used to explain the problem, any reason or assumptions that were used to develop the intervention and reason why the intervention(s) was expected to work" [2].

STUDY OF THE IMPROVEMENT: REPORTING STRENGTH OF EVIDENCE

The effective study of your improvement initiative depends heavily on convincing your reader that the changes that you observed were indeed due to your improvement intervention. Nolan and colleagues have emphasized simply and clearly, "How do you know a change is an improvement? The answer of course is measurement". Such measurement in healthcare improvement requires effective use of appropriate statistical analysis to establish validity and reproducibility [11].

Biomedical scientists are well grounded in parametric statistical methods that we learned in medical or graduate school. Such statistical methodology controls for heterogeneity that is the perceived villain in establishing cause and effect for treatment or diagnostic techniques. On the other hand, in what might appear to be a paradox, it is the richness of this heterogeneity that challenges the healthcare improvement scientist to provide sufficient confidence that a change is indeed an improvement.

Randomized Controlled Trials (RCT)—a bedrock method for many biomedical studies—are extremely useful, but less common in healthcare improvement science for many reasons. The usefulness of the RCT, for example, in the study of a medication for a specific clinical condition comes with all the elegance of simplicity and linearity. Improvement science on the other hand is freighted with the social complexities and heterogeneity that are the stuff of real-world health systems [12]. There are also many practical reasons why the RCT, when it is effectively applied here, is a complicated fit for improvement studies, not the least of which are organizational complexity, time, and cost [13].

Fortunately for our purposes, there are additional statistical methods that serve to validate change, which provide statistically significant confidence in complex social systems over time. Most useful for this purpose is the statistical process control chart. Healthcare improvement science, which has emerged in the late twentieth century, is an adaptation of many statistical methodologies that had their origins in industrial improvement nearly a century earlier. These methodologies were originally championed by the statistician Walter Shewhart at the

Hawthorne Plant of the Western Electric Company in Cicero, IL, in the 1920s and disseminated subsequently principally in manufacturing settings by Shewhart, Joseph Juran, and W. Edwards Deming.

Control charts serve to communicate change that occurs over time with attention to two kinds of variation. The first, common cause variation, is due to chance and is unrelated to an improvement intervention. The second, special cause variation, is identifiable by graphic methods to be unlikely due to chance. While the methodology for control charts is beyond the scope of this book, Coly and Parry provide a useful primer for statistical analysis of complex health interventions [13]. Needless to say, a statistical consultant can be very important to assure that the methodology that you employ is a correct fit.

Be mindful that a convincing report of relevant evidence requires explanation that is understandable and lucid for the statistical non-expert. For this cohort of readers, strive for explicit prose that gives attention to definitions of improvement methodology, specific analyses of data, and a discussion that explains results succinctly and with clarity.

It is reasonable to assume that many of your potential readers may not necessarily be healthcare improvement professionals. Of particular importance to your publication success, these methodologies might be unfamiliar to editors of clinical biomedical journals. As a practical matter, your extra attention to an effective and convincing description of your statistical methodology can benefit from repeated reviews by non-expert colleagues who are willing to test the effectiveness of your explanations.

STUDY OF THE IMPROVEMENT: REPORTING *EX POST* THEORY ANALYSIS

Beyond a clear description of the *prospective* rationale for undertaking an improvement initiative—the "reason-giving" for your initiative in your Introduction—your critical *retrospective ex post* theory analysis of the initiative will greatly strengthen your report. The complexity of this concept has been well developed by Dixon-Woods and colleagues [14] and can be one of the most challenging aspects of reporting healthcare improvement.

Two reports provide lucid and insightful explanations of its complexity [14,15]. The first perspective is provided by a deep dive into layers of context that were associated with the often-cited Keystone Project to Reduce Central Venous Catheter Bloodstream Infections in Intensive Care Units [16]. The second analysis takes ethnographic measurement even further and describes studies associated with the UK Matching Michigan Initiative [15]. Your careful review of these two studies can provide considerable insight into strategies for your retrospective theory development in the report of your improvement initiative.

CASE STUDIES OF *EX POST* THEORY DEVELOPMENT: THE MICHIGAN KEYSTONE PROJECT AND MATCHING MICHIGAN

The analysis of the Michigan Keystone Project to Reduce Central Venous Catheter Bloodstream Infections in Intensive Care Units [16] by Dixon-Woods et al. [14] provides the first vivid example of the value but also the complexity of successful application of critical *ex post* theory development.

Potentially fatal infections associated with deep intravenous catheters were prevalent in most U.S. critical care units in the early twenty-first century. The baseline frequency of up to 5.2 infections per 1000 hours of indwelling venous catheter resulted in an estimated 28,000 deaths annually. A team led by Peter Pronovost proposed testing the effectiveness of an evidence-based strategy for eliminating these complications in intensive care units. They implemented a so-called bundle of acknowledged strategies. It emphasized careful needle insertion technique that included skin sterilization and barrier techniques to keep infection out of the insertion site similar to the technique that a surgeon employs in the operating room. It included regular systematic monitoring of the insertion site and early withdrawal of unnecessary catheters. Initiation of these procedures was nested in changes in the broader unit environment that included a unit-based safety program, clarity about uniform record keeping for tracking infections, hand washing, and tracking clinician-to-clinician communication. These changes were implemented in the great majority of the intensive care units in Michigan. Their report in 2006 [16] described remarkable reduction in morbidity, mortality and cost of care across participating ICUs.

On its face, what more was there to say about this initiative? It remained for Dixon-Woods, in collaboration with Pronovost and colleagues, to plumb further insights that were embedded in this success. How could this outcome be assured in over 100 hospitals that ranged from small community hospitals to large academic medical centers, with diverse levels of expertise and varied local cultures? While it was agreed that the evidence-based bedside techniques were essential to the successful elimination of these infections, these authors retrospectively probed further the details of the social and professional context that led to these successes. To the initial explanations, they re-framed reduction of central line infections as a "social problem...addressing it through a professional movement combining 'grassroots' features with a vertically integrating program structure" [14]. To this they added an emphasis on the horizontal, social, and professional pressures among sites to succeed.

An initiative that was designed to reduce central line infections across healthcare institutions in the United Kingdom was studied by yet another layer of measurement—an extensive ethnographic study of the improvement processes in a sample of participating institutions [15]. This deep analysis involved over 800 hours of observational fieldwork and interviews. It further characterizes the complexity of the data that can constitute accurate assessment of the social context for such a transformative process. To the explanations for the Michigan success, these observations added a very different perspective. They identified wide *variation* across sites, which included the definition of central line infections and which data were obtained and recorded. The pressures to appear effective and safe across comparison institutions were among the subjective *complications* of reporting in these improvement studies.

The work summarized above provides the gold standard for *ex post* theory development. Dixon-Woods and colleagues literally bolted detailed ethnographic and retrospective analyses on the original Keystone and "Matching Michigan" studies. Such a critical analysis of what happened in *your* improvement initiative—and, more importantly, why and how—inevitably can draw on fields beyond traditional biomedical science and includes methodologies more typical of a wide range of social sciences. Bias in data collection across sites, definitions of outcomes that are measured, and technical variation in reporting methods are but a few examples of challenges that can creep into many efforts to improve healthcare [15].

Dixon-Woods goes so far as to describe reports that lack such study as "…distorted imitations that succeed only in reproducing the superficial outer appearance but not the mechanisms… that produced the outcomes in the first instance." This is a blunt reminder that calls for your uncompromising attention.

WHERE DOES *EX POST* THEORY ANALYSIS FIT IN YOUR REPORT?

How can you realistically hope to achieve in your report the level of analysis described in these studies [14,15]? It is fair to say that the remarkable achievements in the original reports from ICUs in Michigan and the United Kingdom were implemented and reported by insightful investigators with analyses of the data that they identified at hand. It is no greater or less than the burden that falls on you as the author of your report.

While *ex post* theory development does not necessarily require the full measure of ethnographic evidence found in the United Kingdom example described by Dixon-Woods [15], it does nevertheless call on you as the author to discern the unfolding of your initiative from every source available. Do not underestimate the place here for astute observations that you have recorded in your journals—real-time observations as the initiative unfolded. Perhaps look back again at the discussion of context in the previous chapter for some of the key elements that others have documented. Your analysis calls for your best application of existing theory to your results, your own deep reflection on as many layers of your context as you can identify. A colleague who is expert in social science methodologies can be an enormously valuable collaborator.

Your decision whether to report this in Results or Discussion, notably in the Limitations summary, requires your candid analysis of how and when such conclusions arose in your initiative. Put your analyses in perspective for your reader by reporting if the social, environmental, or regulatory aspects of the initiative were tracked prospectively. Or rather, might they have become apparent only in retrospect? Your thoughtful reflection serves to lead the reader to important clues to levers as well as hazards for change in their own settings. This critical reflection gets very close to the heart of your improvement work. It provides the principal message for your reader who wants to replicate your success and avoid the pitfalls that you documented.

Recounting these examples of rationale in the CF Network, and *ex post* theory in the Michigan and UK ICU initiatives, emphasizes the complexities of improvement science, particularly reports of large system-wide improvement initiatives. You should be reassured that lessons found in complex, large, system-wide studies such as in these examples that unfold over time—the need for rigorous, consistent tracking of data, the role of theory, ethnographic insights into the complex social settings in which such initiatives are undertaken—are also relevant at the local level [15].

How do you assess how close your manuscript came to providing an accurate report of the study of your improvement initiative? Consider again the value of inviting review by two groups of pre-submission reviewers: first, expert colleagues for methodological validity, and second, non-expert colleagues who might provide the test of understandability of these complex issues for a general reader. The ultimate test for your effectiveness here—I will say it yet again—is how your reader can make effective use of your report for the benefit of further healthcare improvement for their patients and health systems.

In conclusion, the study of your improvement is indeed about much more than simply your description of what happened. The elements that constitute the study of your initiative all call for your attempt to muster the disciplines that are available to you that can buttress your report. Nevertheless, put this daunting task in perspective. Who is more familiar with your work than you, the author? Who better to provide a best effort at describing a rationale, relevant program theory, the strength of evidence, and *ex post* assessment of why your particular initiative was (or was not) successfully implemented?

REFERENCES

1. Davidoff F, Batalden P, Stevens D, The SQUIRE study group. Publication guidelines for quality improvement in health care: Evolution of the SQUIRE project. *Qual Saf Health Care* 2008; (Suppl 1) 17:i3–i9.
2. Ogrinc G, Davies L, Goodman D, et al. SQUIRE 2.0: Revised publication guidelines from a detailed consensus process. *BMJ Qual Saf* 2015;24:466–473.
3. Walshe K. Understanding what works—and why—in quality improvement: The need for theory-driven evaluation. *Int J Qual Health Care* 2007;19(2):57–59.

4. Davidoff F, Dixon-Woods M, Leviton L, et al. Demystifying theory and its use in improvement. *BMJ Qual Saf* 2015;24:228–238.

5. Morgayzel PJ, Dunitz J, Marrow LC, et al. Improving chronic care delivery and outcomes: The impact of the cystic fibrosis care center. *BMJ Qual Saf* 2014;24:i3–i8.

6. Savant AP, Britton LJ, Petren K, et al. Sustained improvement in nutritional outcomes at two pediatric cystic fibrosis centers after quality improvement collaboratives. *BMJ Qual Saf* 2014;24:i81–i89.

7. Savant AP, O'Malley C, Bichl S, et al. Improved patient safety through reduced airway infection rates in a pediatric cystic fibrosis program after a quality improvement effort to enhance infection prevention and control. *BMJ Qual Saf* 2014;24:i73–i80.

8. Zanni RL, Sembrano EU, Du DT, et al. The impact of re-eduction of airway clearance techniques (REACT) on adherence and pulmonary function in patients with cystic fibrosis. *BMJ Qual Saf* 2014;24:i50–i55.

9. Stevens DP, Marshal BC. A decade of improvement in cystic fibrosis: Lessons for other chronic diseases. *BMJ Qual Saf* 2014;24:i1–i2.

10. Pinnock H, Barwick M, Carpenter CR, et al. Standards for reporting implementation studies. *BMJ* 2017;356:i6795. doi:101136/bmj.i6795.

11. Langley GJ, Moen R, Nolan KM, et al. (2009). *The improvement guide: A practical approach to enhancing organizational performance*, 2nd ed. pp. 93–95, San Francisco: Josey-Bass.

12. Davidoff F. Heterogeneity is not always noise: Lessons from improvement. *JAMA* 2009;302:2580–2586.

13. Coly A, Parry G. *Evaluating complex health interventions: A guide to rigorous research designs*. AcademyHealth, 2017. http://www.academyhealth.org/evaluationguide. Accessed September 14, 2107.

14. Dixon-Woods M, Bosk CL, Aveling E-L, et al. Explaining Michigan: Developing an *ex post* theory of a quality improvement program. *Milbank Q* 2011;89:167–205.

15. Dixon-Woods M, Leslie M, Bion J, et al. What counts? An ethnographic study of infection data reported to a patient safety program. *Milbank Q* 2012;90:548–591.

16. Pronovost PD, Needham S, Berenholz D, et al. An intervention to decrease catheter-related bloodstream infections in the ICU. *N Eng J Med* 2006;355:2725–32.

CHAPTER 9

When, where, and how to submit your healthcare improvement manuscript to a journal

IT IS TIME TO SUBMIT YOUR PAPER FOR PUBLICATION

When is your improvement work sufficiently ready to consider submitting your paper to a journal? A therapeutic clinical trial has a defined start and conclusion. On the other hand, an improvement initiative, if it is successful—continuously making a measurable impact on patients' care or the effective and safe function of a health system—may never be truly finished. A useful general rule is, if the changes have been implemented, validated, and established sufficiently, that there is a new normal—in other words, a successful improvement initiative with measurable results—that is an appropriate time to submit your paper for publication.

We have explored how the repeated exposure of a manuscript's drafts to colleagues shares classical principles of improvement—constant small tests and sensible revisions. Ultimately, however, after repeated drafts and re-writes with co-authors, it is time to take the manuscript to the broader world—time to submit the paper to a journal.

SELECT YOUR INTENDED JOURNAL EARLY

Let me step back to try to convince you again that there are efficiencies to be gained by moving your journal selection decision as far forward in time as possible. We previously discussed initiating your draft paper *as you start your improvement initiative*. In addition, move your decision about your intended journal as early in that drafting process as possible.

Authors generally complete a manuscript, and then start the search for a likely journal that might welcome its submission. Instead, there are at least two practical advantages for your *early* selection of a target journal. One is the opportunity to craft your paper's narrative so that it is attentive to tilting the paper's explicit focus toward the journal's likely readership—profession, specialty, etc. The second advantage is that it allows for efficiencies to be found in early attention to that journal's preferred article formats and submission processes.

JOURNALS INCREASINGLY WELCOME HEALTHCARE IMPROVEMENT SUBMISSIONS

Scholarly healthcare improvement reports are found in an increasingly wide-ranging array of journals as healthcare improvement science is recognized to have a broader impact on patient care. The boundaries between healthcare improvement science, implementation science, health services research, and the social sciences are increasingly permeable, and such distinctions are important for you to note in your quest to define potential publication opportunities. In addition, improvement writing for clinical disciplines—for example, surgery, pediatrics, critical care, cardiology, or primary care—requires awareness of the viewpoints that can be found among the respective specialties. This same awareness is useful in your consideration of nursing, pharmacy, or healthcare management readerships.

The good news is that this provides publication opportunities that are created by the convergence of the medical specialties, the related perspectives of healthcare delivery science and health services research. Similar opportunities can be found in nursing and healthcare management. Of greatest importance here is the question of which patients and/ or healthcare systems will benefit the most. This central question leads back yet again to your intended reader.

USE A SYSTEMATIC PROCESS FOR SELECTING A JOURNAL

This leads as well to my encouragement to employ a relatively focused systematic process that includes early selection of your intended journal for submission. Early attention to this decision will influence future decisions as you revise, and thereby provides a greater likelihood that your paper will align with the editorial preferences of your target journal.

Here are five suggested elements developed for a journal selection process that represents a consensus reached by a group of Dartmouth trainee and faculty colleagues. They would be the first to agree that these criteria do not reflect a hard and fast evidence-based consensus, but rather an experience-based suggestion for you and your co-authors to consider.

And please note, there is no need to spend excessive time ruminating on this process. It is pretty simple. Moreover, if you discern a substantial change in any of the journal's selection or other policies listed below as you are drafting and revising your paper, you can readily default to the next journal selection on your list.

1. Start by canvassing your co-authors for suggestions for a list of potential journals that are likely to lead to your intended reader. Take advantage of the special challenges that arise when co-authors are collaborators from diverse disciplines. It offers a wider array of potential journals that are outside your personal experience. Proceed to develop a rank order for consideration.
2. As you winnow this list, start with the basic question, "Why would these readers want to read my intended paper? Is there a fit with these interests?"

3. Now consider several additional pragmatic criteria. Review the instructions to authors for expectations such as adherence to particular publication guidelines, word count, editorial idiosyncrasies that may be reflected by recent changes in editorial leadership or journal ownership. For example, is the journal the organ of a particular specialty society, which might make your paper particularly appealing if your paper targets this field? Scan the journals' associate editors' list for acquaintances who might provide insights into editorial preferences.

4. Based on this background information, narrow your choice to a maximum of three likely candidates. Now scan recent issues for a sense of the current topics, methods, and themes that seem to be of greater interest to the editorial téam. There are gradual trends that can reflect changes over time, so do this early and perhaps once again before submitting.

5. Finally, reach consensus among your co-authors for your intended journal before getting too deeply into the revision process.

JOURNALS THAT WELCOME SCHOLARLY HEALTHCARE IMPROVEMENT SUBMISSIONS

The ever-expanding list of journals that currently welcome healthcare improvement and patient safety submissions can be divided into four groups. Examples are summarized in Table 9.1. The first group of journals is principally focused on healthcare improvement, patient safety, and implementation science topics. They are usually good bets for a welcome review of your well-crafted submission. In addition, there is an expanding second group of journals that, while looking for submissions focused on a broader set of topics, will likely welcome your healthcare improvement submission. The third group consists of clinical specialty journals that increasingly welcome papers that address improvement and patient safety with particular relevance to their specialty readership. Finally, relatively high-impact general journals with broad readerships will bring highly critical reviews to your submission, but increasingly many of these have initiated special sections that are specifically focused on targeted improvement topics.

Table 9.1 A list of representative journals that welcome well-crafted healthcare improvement and patient safety submissions

Journals with principal interest in healthcare improvement science and patient safety
- *BMJ Quality and Safety*, http://qualitysafety.bmj.com/
- *Implementation Science*, https://implementationscience .biomedcentral.com/
- *American Journal of Medical Quality*, https://us.sagepub.com/ en-us/nam/american-journal-of-medical-quality/journal201749
- *Joint Commission Journal on Quality and Patient Safety*, http://www.jointcommissionjournal.com/
- *Journal of Nursing Care Quality*, http://journals.lww.com/ jncqjournal/pages/default.aspx
- *Journal of Patient Safety*, http://journals.lww.com/ journalpatientsafety/pages/default.aspx
- *Circulation Quality and Outcomes*, http://circoutcomes .ahajournals.org/

Journals of broader interests that welcome healthcare improvement science and patient safety
- *The Permanente Journal*, http://www.thepermanentejournal.org /authors.html
- *Milbank Quarterly*, https://www.milbank.org/quarterly/about/
- *Medical Care*, http://journals.lww.com/lww-medicalcare/pages /default.aspx

Consider these journals' specific readerships
- *American Journal of Critical Care*, http://ajcc.aacnjournals.org/
- *Academic Medicine*, http://journals.lww.com/academicmedicine /Pages/currenttoc.aspx
- *Health Affairs*, http://www.healthaffairs.org/
- *Journal of the American College of Surgeons*, http://www .journalacs.org/
- *Pediatrics*, http://pediatrics.aappublications.org /content/140/3?current-issue=y
- *Canadian Journal of Diabetes*, http://www .canadianjournalofdiabetes.com/
- *Critical Care*, https://ccforum.biomedcentral.com/

(Continued)

Table 9.1 (*Continued*) A list of representative journals that welcome well-crafted healthcare improvement and patient safety submissions

- *Annals American Thoracic Society*, http://www.atsjournals.org/journal/annalsats
- *Academic Pediatrics*, http://www.academicpedsjnl.net/

Highest Impact Journals, but worth a try if there is a fit

- *BMJ*, http://www.bmj.com/
- *The Lancet*, http://www.thelancet.com/
- *Annals of Internal Medicine*, http://annals.org/aim
- *New England Journal of Medicine*, http://www.nejm.org/
- *Journal of General Internal Medicine*, http://www.jgim.org/
- *JAMA*, http://jamanetwork.com/journals/jama
- *Canadian Medical Journal*, http://www.cmaj.ca/

EARLY ATTENTION TO SUBMISSION TECHNICALITIES

Once your target journal is selected, pay attention to its formalities and processes for your paper's eventual submission even as you start on your first draft. To assist you with these details, here is a short list of six issues for your early attention. They can help focus your drafting process and free up your later revisions for the important work of sharpening the paper's scholarly messages and refining your writing style.

1. Review carefully the instructions for authors, including attention to format issues that can be as straightforward as hierarchy for section headings, reference style, and table formats.
2. Give early attention to obtaining permission for acknowledgements, personal communications, and reproduced figures. Left to the last minute, these have the potential to introduce frustrating delays that are less troublesome when they appear early in the drafting process.
3. Initiate an early draft of the editor's cover letter so that special requirements are accommodated as the manuscript is revised. Keep your letter brief. Do not hesitate to clearly characterize your opinion of the paper's particular strengths and contributions. Edit your cover letter closely for syntax and clarity—just as closely as you have edited your paper.

4. Accumulate a running list of useful key words or MESH terms that will make the paper particularly accessible to your target readers.
5. Maintain a short list of possible reviewers and their contact information for submission with the paper. Many journals will invite your suggestions of possible reviewers, an opportunity that you do not want to squander. Moreover, even if the journal does not invite suggestions for possible reviewers, you can suggest two or three possible reviewers in your cover letter. Help the editor with this thorny task by providing likely willing volunteers.
6. Finally, use the journal's instructions to authors again as a final checklist before submission. In particular, pay attention to the organization of your paper and abstract.

STEP BACK A MOMENT TO ASSURE YOU HAVE ADDRESSED THE ISSUE OF HUMAN SUBJECTS PROTECTION

Attention to human subjects protection issues is a paramount issue—one of your early tasks in the preparation of your paper for submission. Scholarly journals require assurance that you have obtained institutional oversight of human subjects protection before they consider your paper for publication. Institutional Human Ethics Committees (called Institutional Review Boards [IRBs] in the United States), are charged with the important societal mission of protecting the safety and welfare of human subjects in clinical research [1].

At this point, it is likely that you will have attended to these issues in your initiative as one of the early tasks in anticipation of publication. Nevertheless, here again are suggested strategies for addressing human subjects protection that specifically apply to your improvement initiative.

Human subjects protection review for healthcare improvement initiatives is now generally considered outside the definition of clinical research *per se* (please refer to Chapter 1 for further discussion). Consequently, you have one of two possible approaches for demonstrating evidence of institutional review for your editor. The first is formal IRB approval. It involves your addressing institutional hurdles that include signed patient consent forms similar to those used for clinical research.

A second approach—well worth your consideration as a preferred path—is to meet appropriate criteria for a formal waiver by the committee. Generally, ethics committees and staff will define for you the process for meeting the requirements for such a waiver [2]. Take advantage of their explicit advice regarding the formal process.

Keep in mind as you negotiate with your IRB that, traditionally, many local IRBs considered healthcare improvement studies to be human subjects clinical research. It will be important to make the case to your IRB explicitly that your improvement initiative does not involve experimental therapy, but rather the implementation of a variation on "usual care." A substantial part of the argument that makes this case is that if the change were left unimplemented, it would result in a poorer standard of care for all patients [1,2]. Most editors will consider notification of a formal waiver from your IRB as sufficient to meet their obligation to assure human subjects protection. Make ample use of the advice by Ogrinc et al. [2] as you approach this negotiation.

TAKE FULL ADVANTAGE OF THE JOURNAL'S REVIEW PROCESS

Return now to the formal manuscript submission process. You will be expected to use your journal's online submission site, for example, ScholarOne. Each site has its own technical processes that you will follow for your submission, and there is little room for deviation. If you are new to the site, you will find an introductory set of instructions that provides guidance for navigation of the submission process as you walk through a series of download and/or cut-and-paste activities. Generally, plan to set aside 2–3 hours for undistracted computer time online to complete your submission.

Ultimately, the journal's initial review process is straightforward and is in the hands of the editor and editorial staff. It is reasonable to expect fair and prompt reviews. The editor sits at the hub of the review process while the reviewers provide advice to the editor in their formal reviews and recommendations.

There are at least two processes that can slow down your review. The first is the universal challenge that most journals encounter—finding willing reviewers. The second is the reviewers' time for squeezing review of your paper into their busy professional lives.

In any event, in spite of the editor's best intentions, delays can occur. Be mindful that the editor navigates this same process with scores of papers. Should it seem to you that your paper is languishing past the journal's published turn-around time for review, it is reasonable for you to send a short note requesting an update on the paper's progress. A reasonable time limit before contacting the editor is 2–4 weeks beyond the journal's published review time.

When the initial review process is completed, the editor will collate the reviewers' opinions and communicate them to you with conclusions and recommendations. If the editor indicates that the journal will consider your paper for possible publication, the decision will probably be accompanied by detailed requests for changes in your paper. This puts you and your co-authors back at the center of the process. Move promptly to this stage of your work.

Strategic use of the review and revision process will invariably lead to the best possible final published article. A long list of detailed reviewers' comments for changes in your paper may appear daunting. In your response, acknowledge in exquisite detail their comments, point by point. Most importantly, respond to each and every reviewer's comments and refer explicitly to the place in your manuscript where you have made appropriate changes.

As you peruse the detailed comments, be mindful that your reviewers will have contributed substantially to the improvement of your paper when they offer suggestions for refining your paper—on average at least 5–7 hours of their time. Develop your response to the editor promptly.

This revision with your co-authors is a complicated activity that calls for diplomacy, coordination, and cooperation. It is a negotiation that never follows the same path. As first author, it is a good idea to frame a tentative revision strategy before you approach your co-authors. Proceed to systematically examine the comments with all your co-authors. Divide up the reviewers' comments for responses among your co-authors. Journal reviews can sometimes be the source of bruised egos among your co-authors, which might require your counsel. The final response to your editor still ultimately comes down to you as first author to collate the responses and the revised draft. Your paper might proceed through several revisions. Do not assume its acceptance until you receive the editor's formal acceptance notice.

There are two potentially thorny issues that might arise requiring your response outside the usual revise and resubmit process. First, uncommonly, you may believe there has been a misunderstanding by a reviewer. It is appropriate to state this explicitly and diplomatically in the communication that accompanies your revision.

Second, if you believe there is bias reflected in a review that should disqualify the reviewer, you should communicate directly with the editor. But first, test your response with a trusted colleague or mentor to assure your own measure of objectivity.

It is both reassuring and useful to remember that should this editor reject your paper, that rejection can be a valuable part of the improvement process on the way to its eventual publication—a fact that is often difficult to acknowledge when the rejection letter first arrives. The editor will usually communicate all the reviewers' comments to you, and often offer valuable advice as you consider submission to another journal.

On a rare occasion, you may consider it reasonable to ask the editor to consider an appeal to the rejection—accompanied by a brief outline of the explicit issues on which you base your appeal. It rarely works, so appeal only if you believe you have a strong case. Allow a sufficient interval for bruised egos to heal, but then it is time to buckle down to the work of repeating the submission process with your next candidate journal.

YOUR ROLE AFTER PUBLICATION

If your paper has been accepted for publication, congratulations! The improvement author's task is not finished when the paper is published. Reflect again on the overriding goal for your writing and publishing—your paper's contribution to improving healthcare. This calls for a series of additional tasks—a comprehensive dissemination strategy for this new knowledge.

It is appropriate for you to bring your paper's publication to the attention of colleagues. For example, share your good news in department meetings. Communicate widely with colleagues in your field.

It serves the improvement process for your institutional leadership to be aware of your paper and its reflection on the institution's commitment to patient care improvement and safety. Editors and publishers generally encourage the author to contact institutional public affairs officials. Consider an Op Ed piece for your local news sources. Be prepared to frame your message for a lay audience—a brief, useful message that is not burdened by jargon. And, of course, do not overstate the paper's message.

CONSIDER A BROADER PUBLICATION STRATEGY

As you and your co-authors celebrate your successful publication, consider yet another set of tasks—the development of a broader publication strategy that can serve to amplify the impact of your initial improvement findings. For example, the breadth of your initiative's results might suggest opportunities for several additional papers. To avoid potential misunderstandings or conflicts as the work unfolds, make early and explicit decisions among your co-authors with clarity about authorship, deliverables, and deadlines. An example is a systematic review that is based on the literature scan that led to the initiative. Another is a commentary that expands on the work's relevance and its potential impact for specific clinical disciplines represented by your co-authors. Consider your article's publication as only the beginning of the next steps in the improvement process.

A FEW FINAL OBSERVATIONS ABOUT YOUR SUCCESSFUL PUBLICATION

It is not surprising that authors often see scholarly publication as the navigation of a difficult path between authors and investigators on the one hand, and editors and reviewers on the other. In fact, editors and reviewers share your success when your paper is published.

The International Committee of Medical Journal Editors (ICMJE) proposes a thoughtful, pragmatic view for a larger context for the place for editorial peer review in scholarly publication. In *Recommendations for Conduct, Reporting, Editing and Publication of Scholarly Work in Medical Journals*, the ICMJE suggests that *valid* peer review might actually only begin with the formal publication of the work [3]. The implication of this high-level theory is that postpublication interaction among colleagues provides the true measure of the paper's fit with the scholarly work that both preceded it but *also that inevitably follows* as time unfolds. This larger context has been facilitated by the emerging role for electronic media in scholarly publication. Consider this perspective—peer review writ large—as you contemplate the place for your paper in the larger healthcare improvement community.

REFERENCES

1. Lynn J, Baily MA, Bottrell M, et al. The ethics of using quality improvement methods in health care. *Ann Intern Med* 2007;146:666–673.

2. Ogrinc G, Nelson WA, Adams SM, et al. An instrument to differentiate between clinical research and quality improvement. *IRB* 2013;35:1–8.
3. International Committee of Medical Journal Editors. Recommendations for the conduct, reporting, editing, and publication of scholarly work in medical journals. Updated December 2016. http://www.icmje.org/icmje-recommendations.pdf. Accessed September 9, 2017.

APPENDIX
A comprehensive writing curriculum for trainees*

BACKGROUND

Medical, nursing, and health management training programs that include healthcare improvement and patient safety in their curricula should place a high priority on scholarly publication. This is based on the principle that healthcare improvement is incomplete until it is published. Trainees' successful publication can be achieved by a formal program that is designed to develop their writing competence.

Such a formal writing initiative for trainees and faculty has been part of the Dartmouth Leadership and Preventive Medicine Residency (LPMR) since its inception. The LPMR provides examples of useful curricula for such an initiative.

RATIONALE FOR A TRAINEE WRITING CURRICULUM

The overarching rationale for a comprehensive trainee writing curriculum is the integration of excellent scholarly writing for publication into the trainee's work of healthcare improvement. Writing and successful publication

---

* Adapted from The Dartmouth–Hitchcock Leadership and Preventive Medicine Residency Scholarly Writing Collaborative

occupy a central place in a successful career in healthcare improvement. Importantly, the reflective nature of writing offers insights into the author's work and identity that can lead to deeper professional insight.

A CULTURE THAT STRESSES THE EXPECTATION OF SCHOLARLY PUBLICATION

There are two overarching elements that constitute such a program. First among them is a *program culture that places unequivocal emphasis on scholarly publication*. Such a culture places a collective obligation on a community of improvement scholars to share responsibility for successful publication.

Accordingly, a community of healthcare improvement scholars, at its best, supports each other's creative work of writing and publication and should aim collectively to write with the greatest clarity. Writing, reviewing, and revising at their most effective are processes where colleagues are constantly assisting each other to achieve transparency and clarity of expression so that ultimately a colleague's research, by its publication, is most accessible to his/her colleagues.

Each trainee is expected to prepare one or more publications based on his or her improvement research. Diverse LPMR trainee clinical and academic backgrounds dictated explicit attention to residents' variable writing experience. Faculty participants served as important role models for the professional habit of writing and co-learners in scholarly writing. The LPMR found that a monthly scholarly writing session—with an associated commitment by faculty, and expectation of resident preparation—established the explicit expectation for regular scholarly writing as a component of healthcare improvement.

PEER REVIEW AT EVERY STAGE OF THE WRITING PROGRAM

Peer review is the second essential element for a program that helps trainees achieve critical scholarly publication. Accordingly, LPMR trainees and faculty developed explicit rules and strategies for effective peer review as a skill linked to productive writing. Meeting one afternoon a month, participants generally write, working in pairs alternating as either author or reviewer.

The hierarchy across attending physicians and resident trainees is leveled when trainees and faculty meet to write together. While faculty members are usually more experienced writers, few find writing for publication easy. Similarly, faculty find the process of sharing early drafts daunting, which contributes to a leveling of the hierarchy among learners.

ORGANIZING PRINCIPLES

Trainees should:

1. Incorporate writing as an integral part of their work in healthcare improvement and patient safety.
2. Understand the scholarly peer-review and editorial processes.
3. Improve writing competence.
4. Publish at least one scholarly peer-reviewed paper.

Faculty Coaches will:

1. Model by their own writing the work of successful scholarly writing.
2. Participate as co-learners with trainees in monthly writing sessions.
3. Work actively with trainees as writing coaches and co-authors, helping to move their work to successful publication.

Faculty coaches provide prominent role models for trainees. They serve as active participants, both in class discussion but also as coaches and mentors for residents as they move their papers through drafts to submission.

Self-assessment surveys that have been administered to successive cohorts of trainees consistently demonstrate wide heterogeneity of writing experience and serve to align learning strategies with participants' competence. Prior writing experience for most residents is usually associated with clinical activities. A minority of LPMR residents had participated in research electives as students or residents, which had led to contributions as a co-author to formal biomedical publications.

Each participant will commit to preparation and submission of one or more scholarly papers during their training program. These papers will be linked to their individual improvement work and will also take advantage of assignments for other aspects of the trainee's course work. For example, preparation of a systematic literature review for one component of the program might serve effectively as the basis for a paper for submission to a peer-reviewed journal.

Trainees' writing should progress in tandem with their research: at each stage of the author's work, the emerging manuscript will reflect the status of the work's implementation and results as they fit into a research paper. Early on, for example, the Introduction of the research report might reflect the systematic literature review. The Methods will reflect the evolution of the project's interventions. A draft Discussion might anticipate a theory of the expected outcomes, and will inevitably evolve over time. In sum, writing activities in the course are intended to provide synergy and leverage for both formal course work and an improvement project.

Formal publication guidelines can offer a framework for the curriculum depending on the curriculum topic for a particular session. For example, class discussion can be anchored in the SQUIRE 2.0 Publication Guidelines (Standards for Quality Improvement Reporting Excellence), StaRI as a checklist for elements of implementation science reports, or PRISMA for systematic reviews.

Trainees and faculty meet formally for 2–4 hours every month. Evaluation for the LPMR program is based on both participation and quality of writing. Fifty percent is based on class attendance and participation, and fifty percent is based on scholarly productivity. First and second year trainees frequently meet as separate cohorts with course faculty to address writing priorities that address the respective stages of professional development represented by the two cohorts.

TEN SESSIONS FOR A TRAINEE WRITING PROGRAM

Session 1: Getting started and keeping going with your writing

Overview:
    The collaborative will start with a course outline, aims, and proposed pedagogy.

1. The writing collaborative, its aims and objectives will be reviewed.
   a.   Unique elements of scholarly writing to improve healthcare
   b.   Getting started and keeping going in one's writing
   c.   The use of writing as a reflective activity
2. Participants will reflect on their own expectations for the writing collaborative, their writing strengths, and the opportunities for improvement.
3. The program will emphasize integration of one's scholarly writing into one's daily improvement work.
4. Participants will serve as both authors and reviewers.
5. Why a writing collaborative is important to the work of improvement.
6. Why it's a challenge to share work in progress, etc.
7. Titles.

Pre-work:

1. Prepare a personal writing self-assessment and come to class prepared to reflect on relating your self-assessment to your learning goals.
2. Review the Table of Contents of three issues of a clinical journal that you generally read. What titles attract your interest? Why? What are the characteristics of effective titles? Of less effective titles?
3. Develop a draft title for your own work in progress.

Self-assessment survey:
   The following questions are intended to guide your reflection on your scholarly writing activities, areas for personal improvement, and your expectations for this Workshop.

1. Proposed paper or topic (draft working title, if available)
2. How often do you actually sit down and write for scholarly purposes?
3. When and where do you write?
4. How many scholarly (peer-reviewed) papers of any kind have you published?
5. What do you consider your strengths in scholarly writing?
6. What are your objectives for your participation in this Workshop?

Session 2: An introduction to the role of publication guidelines in your writing

Overview:

1. IMRaD (Introduction, Methods, Results, and Discussion) as a framework
2. Publication Guidelines
3. The study aim

Participants will examine the rationale and substance of two scholarly publication guidelines, particularly as they apply to healthcare improvement and patient safety research. The guidelines field will be scanned, but the principal focus will be on SQUIRE 2.0 (Standards for QUality Improvement Excellence) and PRISMA (Preferred Reporting Items for Systematic Reviews and Meta-Analyses). The session specifically will address framing the study aim. Participants will present their own examples and use the opportunity to explore how careful attention to framing the aim serves both the improvement research and its scholarly publication.

Pre-work:

1. Review SQUIRE 2.0 and PRISMA Publication Guidelines.
2. Participants will prepare a statement of their project aim, as they would write it for publication.

Readings:

1. Holzmueller CG, Pronovost PJ. Organising a manuscript reporting quality improvement or patient safety research. *BMJ Qual Saf* 2013;22:777–785.
2. Ogrinc G, Davies L, Goodman D, et al. SQUIRE 2.0 (Standards for QUality Improvement Excellence): Revised publication guidelines from a detailed consensus process. *BMJ Qual Saf* 2016;25(12):986–992.
3. Moher D, Liberati A, Tetzlaff J, et al. The PRISMA Group. Preferred reporting items for systematic reviews and meta-analyses: The PRISMA statement. *PLoS Med.* 2009;6(7):e1000097. PMID: 19621072.

Session 3: What format is appropriate for your paper?

Overview:

This session focuses on the broader scholarly healthcare improvement literature. First, we will explore opportunities that are presented by short reports, with particular attention to case reports of improvement as reflected in Quality Improvement Reports (QIR). Then, we relate QIRs to the broader improvement literature.

Objectives:

1. Examine the place for case reports—with focus on Quality Improvement Reports (QIR)—in the broader scholarly improvement literature. How are QIRs similar or different from clinical case reports?
2. Review the opportunities for short pithy contributions to the scholarly improvement literature, including a run at framing a brief QIR.
3. Develop practical strategies for approaching editors for reports other than original comprehensive improvement research reports.
4. Explore published views of the current scholarly improvement literature.
5. Build a draft typology of the improvement literature for personal use when considering submission of work for publication.

Pre-work:

Please review the Moss and Thomson description of Quality Improvement Report (QIR) guidelines and the Vandenbroucke paper on clinical case reports. Please reflect on your perspective of the utility of brief case reports in the scholarly improvement literature. How can that utility and value be enhanced?

Readings:

1. Moss F, Thomson R. A new structure for quality improvement reports. *Qual Saf Health Care* 2004;13:6–7.
2. Vandenbroucke JP. In defense of case reports and case series. *Ann Intern Med* 2001;134:330–334.
3. Stevens DP. The context is the "news" in healthcare improvement case reports. *Qual Saf Health Care* 2010;19:162–163.

Session 4: Increasing writing efficiency; making your paper accessible to your reader

Overview:

1. Defining a time and a place to write.
2. Explore the importance of making your writing accessible to your reader: Title and Abstract.
3. Learn strategies for raising the visibility of your work by addressing how readers approach an article.

Pre-work:

1. Reflect on when and where you write.
2. Participants will continue work on a title.
3. Draft an abstract and conclusion for a work in progress.
4. Develop six key words for your work.

Readings:

1. Neuhauser D, McEachern E, Zyzanski S, et al. Continuous quality improvement and the process of writing for academic publications. *Qual Manag Health Care* 2000;8:65–73.
2. Holzmueller CE, Pronovost PJ. Organizing a manuscript reporting quality improvement or patient safety research. *BMJ Qual Saf* 2013;22:777–785.

Session 5: Reviewing, editing and the author

Overview:

1. Gain facility with critiquing manuscripts for scholarly journals.
2. Develop key points for a review.
3. Understand how initial manuscripts may be modified by the review process.
4. Relate this reviewing experience to one's own work as an author.

Pre-work:

1. Read Richard Smith's perspective of peer review and reflect on how this relates to your use of peer review to improve your draft manuscript.
2. Review *Proposed Elements of a Successful Review.* How might you modify this approach?

Proposed elements of a successful review:

1. As a rule, identify the reviewer's competence to review this particular paper.
2. Be mindful of any potential conflict of interest.
3. Be specific.
4. Prioritize advice.
5. Systematically read the *entire* paper (or the draft parts for review).
6. Identify the best fit for this paper in the literature.
7. Summarize explicit strengths and weaknesses.
8. Cite sections with opportunities for improvement accompanied by appropriate, specific suggestions.
9. Examine carefully the tables and figures for clarity, relevance, ease of reading, legends, and how the author fits them into the narrative.
10. Is the paper complete? What is missing?
11. Where appropriate, make use of a brief content checklist (*see SQUIRE 2.0 Publication Guidelines*) for inclusion of:
    a. An explicit improvement aim and study question
    b. Description of the intervention in sufficient detail that others might reproduce it in their settings
    c. Description of the study design (for example, observational, quasi-experimental, experimental) chosen for measuring the impact of the intervention on outcomes
    d. Report of results that appear valid as well as meaningful to a broad readership
    e. Conclusion regarding the implications of this work for patients and/or systems of care

Readings:

1. Jefferson T, Wager E, Davidoff F. Measuring the quality of editorial peer review. *JAMA* 2002;287:2786–2790.
2. Smith R. Peer review: A flawed process at the heart of science and journals. *J R Soc Med* 2006;99:178–182.

Session 6: Context

Overview:

1. This session will focus on "Context" and its important role in writing for the scholarly improvement literature.
2. Explore the importance of "Context" in reporting improvement work.
3. Examine the utility of SQUIRE publication guidelines for communicating "Context."
4. Recognize differences between setting and context.
5. Postulate relevant contextual elements in your own improvement initiative.

Pre-work:

1. Review Taylor et al. and Kaplan et al. as summaries of contextual elements in healthcare improvement reports.
2. For orientation, review again how "Context" is addressed by the SQUIRE 2.0 Guidelines.
3. Review again Batalden and Davidoff's classic article from 2007, What is "quality improvement" and how can it transform health care.

Readings:

1. Stevens DP. The context is the "news" in healthcare improvement case reports. *Qual Saf Health Care* 2010;19:162–163.
2. Taylor SL, Dy S, Foy R, Hempel S, et al. What context features might be important determinants of the effectiveness of patient safety interventions? *BMJ Qual Saf* 2011;20:611–617.

3. Batalden PB, Davidoff F. What is "quality improvement" and how can it transform health care. *Qual Saf Health Care* 2007;16:2–3.
4. Kaplan HC, Brady PW, Dritz MC, et al. The influence of context on improvement success in Health Care: A systematic review of the literature. *Milbank Q* 2010;88:500–559.
5. Stevens DP, Shojania KG. Tell me about the context, and more. *BMJ Qual Saf* 2011;20:557–559.

Session 7: Rationale

Overview:

1. This session will focus on describing the Rationale for your improvement initiative.
2. Examine challenges of communicating Rationale prospectively and an ex post explanation of why and how an initiative worked.

Pre-work:

1. Read Davidoff et al. for a process in developing the Rationale for your initiative ("If…, then…, so that… etc.").
2. How does a prospective Rationale differ from an ex post theory analysis as characterized by Dixon-Woods, et al.?

Readings:

1. Walshe K. Understanding what works—and why—in quality improvement: The need for theory-driven evaluation. *Int J Qual Health Care* 2007;19(2):57–59.
2. Davidoff F, Dixon-Woods M, Leviton L, et al. Demystifying theory and its use in improvement. *BMJ Qual Saf* 2015;24: 228–238.
3. Dixon-Woods M, Bosk CL, Aveling EL, et al. Explaining Michigan: Developing an *ex post* theory of a quality improvement program. *Milbank Q* 2011;89:167–205.
4. Dixon-Woods M, Leslie M, Bion J, et al. What counts? An ethnographic study of infection data reported to a patient safety program. *Milbank Q* 2012;90:548–591.

Session 8: Working with coauthors

Overview:

1. "If you can't describe what you're doing as a process, you don't know what you're doing." W. Edwards Deming insisted that effective work should be defined as a process. The session will explore strategies for working effectively with co-authors as a process.
2. How might the process of working with co-authors take advantage of Microsystem principles?

Pre-work:

Review The Task of Coauthors: A consensus summary developed by the Dartmouth-Hitchcock LPMR Writing Initiative. How would you modify this approach?

The Task of Coauthors:

1. Identify purpose for each person and maintain clarity of each role as reflected in the author order.
2. Identify the shared investments in the project.
3. Be clear about each person's strengths and weaknesses.
4. Verbalize respect for each other but reflect brutal honesty.
5. Complement/compliment each other.
6. Give and receive feedback effectively.
7. Practice being an outsider – bring fresh eyes to the work.
8. Hold own products lightly.
9. Establish consensus about the aim of the paper.
10. Agree upon structure and timeline for the work.
11. Develop appropriate and effective communication.
12. Be clear about how decisions are made.
13. Maintain momentum in the writing.
14. Respect time/space/boundaries/timeliness.
15. Use all resources.

Readings:

1. Neuhauser D, McEachern E, Zyzanski S, et al. Continuous quality improvement and the process of writing for academic publications. *Qual Manag Health Care* 2000;8:65–73.

2. Nelson EC, Batalden PB, Huber TP, et al. Microsystems in health care: Part 1. Learning from high-performing frontline clinical units. *Joint Comm J Qual Saf*;28:472–493.

Session 9: Writing style: An exercise in close reading

Overview:
    The session will focus on close reading of exemplary authors as a strategy to develop elements of an effective writing style. What are your criteria for inclusion?

Pre-work:

1. Reflect on your favorite scholarly authors. Consider the characteristics that led to inclusion in such a list.
2. What are examples of what you consider their interesting, memorable scholarly writing?

Readings:

1. Charon R. Narrative Medicine. Honoring the Stories of Illness. New York: Oxford University Press. 2006. Particularly see pp 52–53, and pp 114–127.
2. Klinkenborg V. Several short sentences about writing. New York: Alfred A. Knopf. 2012. 204 pp.
3. *AMA Manual of Style. A Guide for Authors and Editors* (JAMA editors and staff) Oxford University Press, 2007 (10th edition).
4. *Writing Science in Plain English* (Anne E. Greene) University of Chicago Press, 2013.
5. *The Craft of Scientific Communication* (Joseph E. Harmon and Alan G. Gross) University of Chicago Press, 2010.

Session 10: Putting it all together: Where to submit your paper?

Overview:

1. Review trainees' draft papers that are in preparation for publication.
2. Gain further experience as reviewer and/or author.
3. Probe the challenges of writing for public discussion.

4. Develop strategies that take one's writing beyond formula and stereotype.
5. What is an appropriate journal for your proposed report?

Pre-work:

Participants will submit a current draft paper for discussion. These can be at any stage of development, not necessarily the completed paper. The group will focus on two or three working drafts, initially in small groups, and then as the entire group.

Readings:

1. International Committee of Medical Journal Editors. Recommendations for the conduct, reporting, editing, and publication of scholarly work in medical journals. Updated December 2016. http://www.icmje.org/icmje-recommendations.pdf. Accessed September 9, 2017.

Index

Printed in the United States
by Baker & Taylor Publisher Services